Ultimate Anti Inflammatory Diet Cookbook

Quick and Easy Meat Recipes to Effortless your Health

Zac Gibson

Table of Contents

Party Chicken Tenders

Prep Time:
25 minutes
Serve: 4

Ingredients:

- ¾ pound chicken tenders
- Prep + Cook Time2 whole eggs, beaten
- ½ cup seasoned breadcrumbs
- ½ cup all-purpose flour
- 1 tbsp black pepper
- 2 tbsp olive oil

Directions:

1.Preheat your air fryer to 330 F. Add breadcrumbs, eggs and flour in three separate bowls (individually).

2.Mix breadcrumbs with oil and season with salt and pepper.

3.Dredge the tenders into flour, eggs and the crumbs.

4.Add chicken tenders in the Air Fryer and cook for 10 minutes. Increase to 390 F, and cook for 5 more minutes.

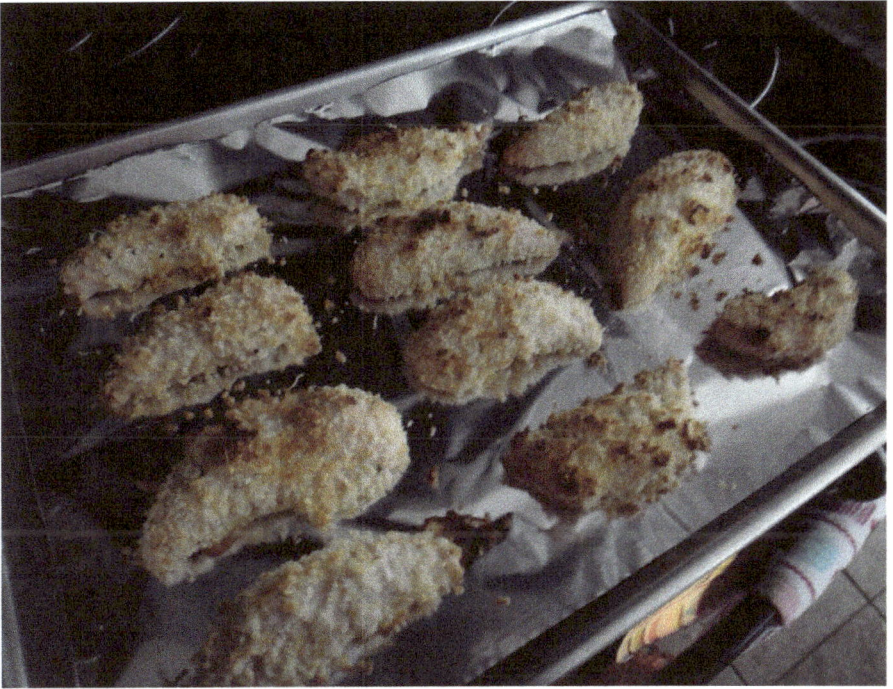

Chicken Tenders with Pineapple Juice

Prep Time:
4h 15 minutes
Serve: 4

Ingredients:

- 1 lb boneless and skinless chicken tenders
- 4 cloves garlic, chopped
- 4 scallions, chopped
- 2 tbsp sesame seeds, toasted
- 1 tbsp fresh ginger, grated
- ½ cup pineapple juice
- ½ cup soy sauce
- ⅓ cup sesame oil
- A pinch of black pepper

Directions:

1.Skew each tender and trim any excess fat. Mix the other ingredients in one large bowl.

2.Add the skewered chicken and place in the fridge for 4 to 24 hours. Preheat the Air Fryer to 375°F.

3.Using a paper towel, pat the chicken until it is completely dry. Fry for 10 minutes.

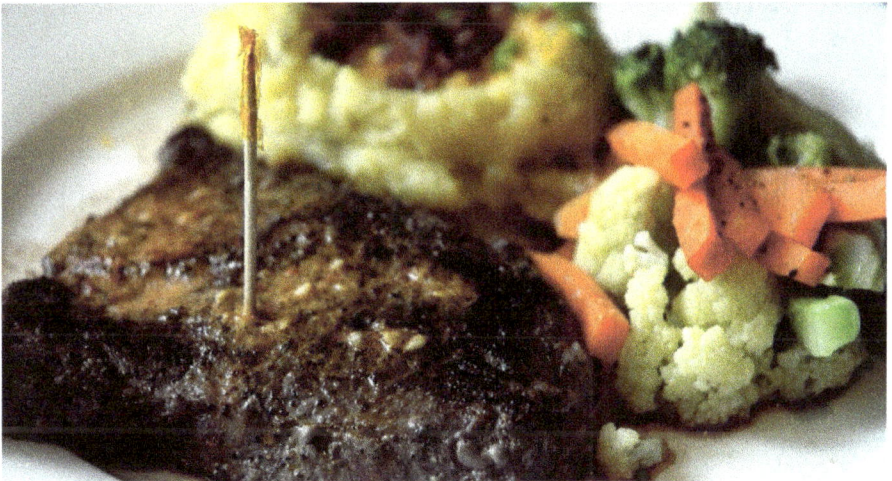

Crispy Panko Turkey Breasts

Prep Time:
25 minutes
Serve: 6

Ingredients:

- 3 turkey breasts, boneless and skinless
- 2 cups panko1 tbsp salt
- ½ tsp cayenne pepper
- ½ tbsp black pepper
- 1 stick butter, melted

Directions:

1.In a bowl, combine the panko, half of the black pepper, cayenne pepper, and half of the salt.

2.In another small bowl, combine the melted butter with salt and pepper. Don't add salt if you use salted butter.

3.Brush the butter mixture over the turkey breasts. Coat the turkey with the panko mixture.

4.Arrange them on a lined baking dish.

5.Air fry for 15 minutes at 390 degrees F. If the turkey breasts are thinner, cook only for 8 minutes.

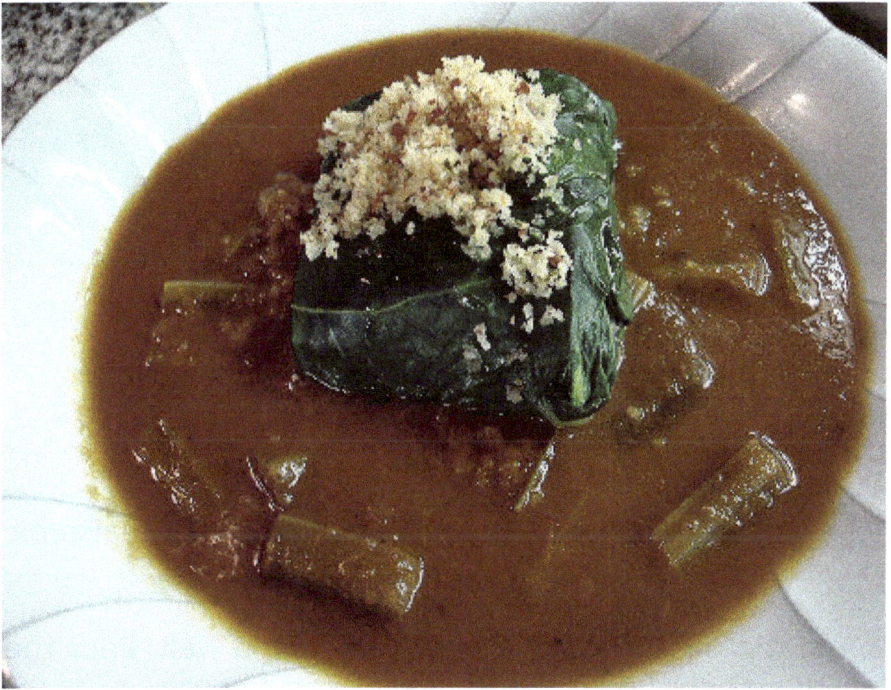

Avocado-Mango Chicken Breasts

Prep Time:
3 hrs 20 minutes
Serve: 2

Ingredients:

- 2 chicken breasts, cubed
- 1 large mango, cubed
- 1 medium avocado, sliced
- 1 red pepper, chopped
- 5 tbsp balsamic vinegar
- 15 tbsp olive oil
- 4 garlic cloves, minced
- 1 tbsp oregano
- 1 tbsp parsley, chopped
- A pinch of mustard powder
- Salt and black pepper to taste

Directions:

1.In a bowl, mix whole mango, garlic, oil, and balsamic vinegar.

2.Add the mixture to a blender and blend well. Pour the liquid over chicken cubes and soak for 3 hours.

3.Take a pastry brush and rub the mixture over breasts as well.

4.Preheat your Air Fryer to 360 F. Place the chicken cubes in the cooking basket, and cook for 12 minutes.

5.Add avocado, mango and pepper and toss well. Drizzle balsamic vinegar and garnish with chopped parsley.

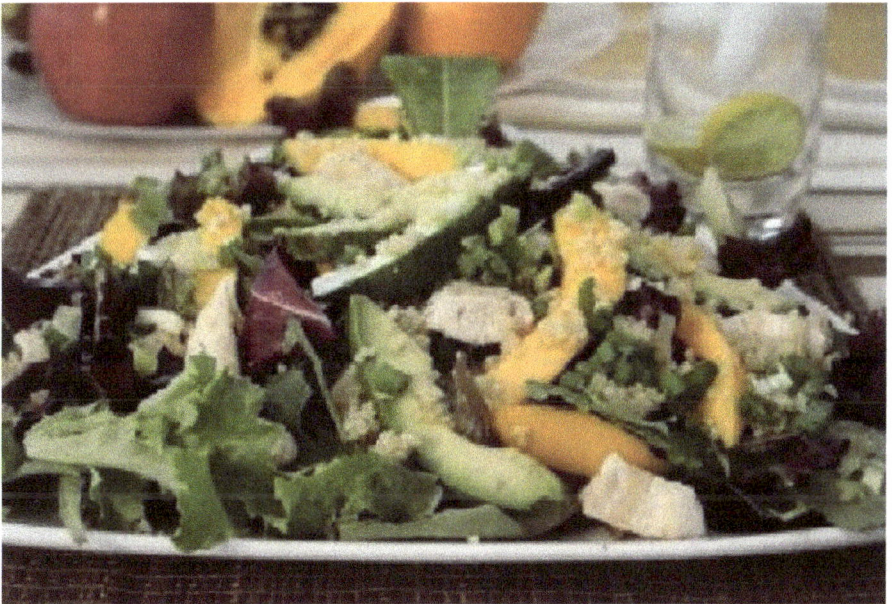

Turkey Nuggets with Parsley & Thyme

Prep Time:
20 minutes
Serve: 2

Ingredients:

- 8 oz turkey breast, boneless and skinless
- 1 egg, beaten
- 1 cup breadcrumbs
- 1 tbsp dried thyme
- ½ tbsp dried parsley
- Salt and black pepper to taste

Directions:

1.Preheat the air fryer to 350 F. Mince the turkey in a food processor; transfer to a bowl.

2.Stir in the thyme and parsley, and season with salt and pepper.

3.Take a nugget-sized piece of the turkey mixture and shape it into a ball, or another form.

4.Dip in the breadcrumbs, then egg, then in the breadcrumbs again.

5.Place the nuggets onto a prepared baking dish, and cook for 10 minutes.

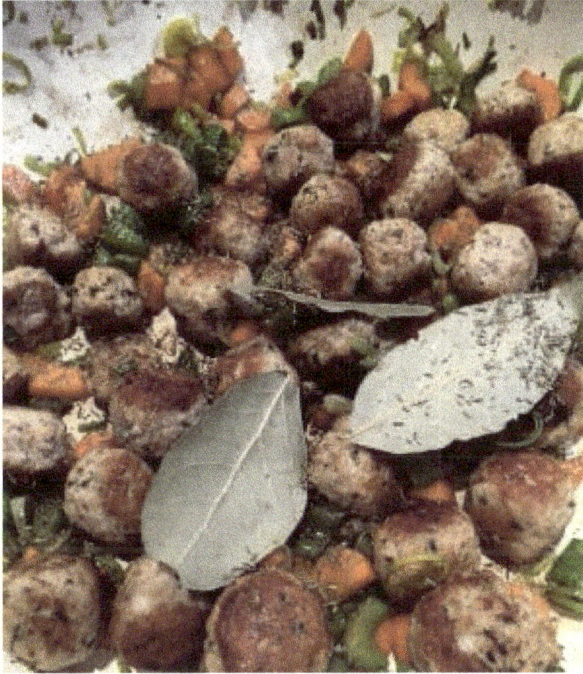

Korean-Style Honey Chicken Wings

Prep Time:
15 minutes
Serve: 5

Ingredients:

- 1 pound chicken wings
- 8 oz flour
- 8 oz breadcrumbs
- 3 beaten eggs
- 4 tbsp Canola oil
- Salt and black pepper to taste
- 2 tbsp sesame seeds
- 2 tbsp Korean red pepper paste
- 1 tbsp apple cider vinegar
- 2 tbsp honey
- 1 tbsp soy sauce
- Sesame seeds, to serve

Directions:

1.Separate the chicken wings into winglets and drumettes. In a bowl, mix salt, oil and pepper.

2.Preheat your Air Fryer to a temperature of 350 F. Coat the chicken with beaten eggs followed by breadcrumbs and flour.

3.Place the chicken in your Air Fryer's cooking basket.

4.Spray with a bit of oil and cook for 15 minutes.

5.Mix red pepper paste, apple cider vinegar, soy sauce, honey and ¼ cup of water in a saucepan and bring to a boil over medium heat. Transfer the chicken to sauce mixture and toss to coat. Garnish with sesame to enjoy!

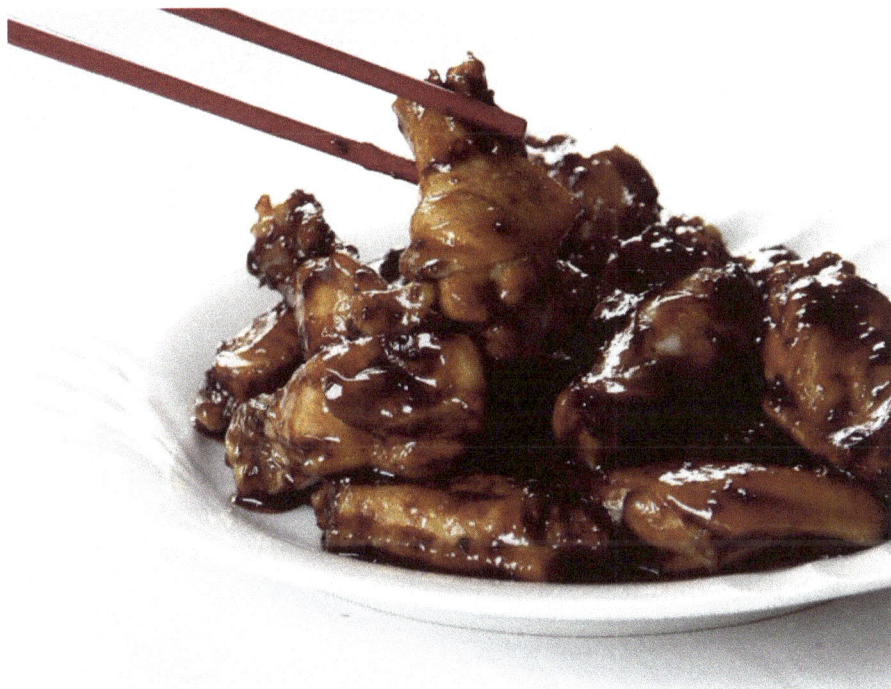

Savory Chicken Drumsticks with Honey and Garlic

Prep Time:
20 minutes
Serve: 3

Ingredients:

- 2 chicken drumsticks, skin removed
- 2 tbsp olive oil
- 2 tbsp honey
- ½ tbsp garlic, minced

Directions:

1.Preheat your Air Fryer to 400 F.

2.Add garlic, oil and honey to a sealable zip bag.

3.Add chicken and toss to coat; set aside for 30 minutes.

4.Add the coated chicken to the Air Fryer basket, and cook for 15 minutes.

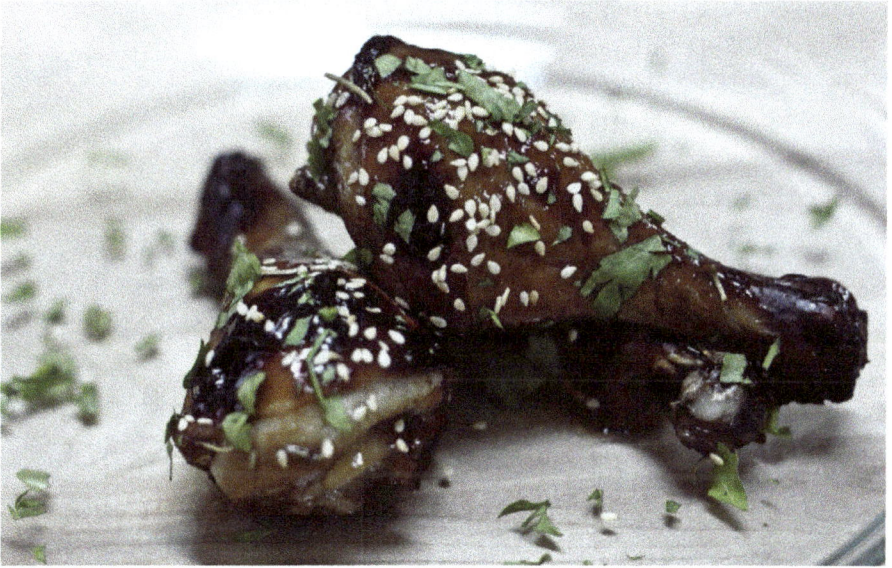

Garlic-Buttery Chicken Wings

Prep Time:
20 minutes
Serve: 4

Ingredients:

- 16 chicken wings
- ¼ cup butter
- ¼ cup honey
- ½ tbsp salt
- 4 garlic cloves, minced
- ¾ cup potato starch

Directions:

1.Preheat the air fryer to 370 F. Rinse and pat dry the wings, and place them in a bowl.

2.Add the starch to the bowl, and mix to coat the chicken.

3.Place the chicken in a baking dish that has been previously coated with cooking oil.

4.Cook for 5 minutes in the air fryer. Whisk the rest of the ingredients together in a bowl.

5.Pour the sauce over the wings and cook for another 10 minutes.

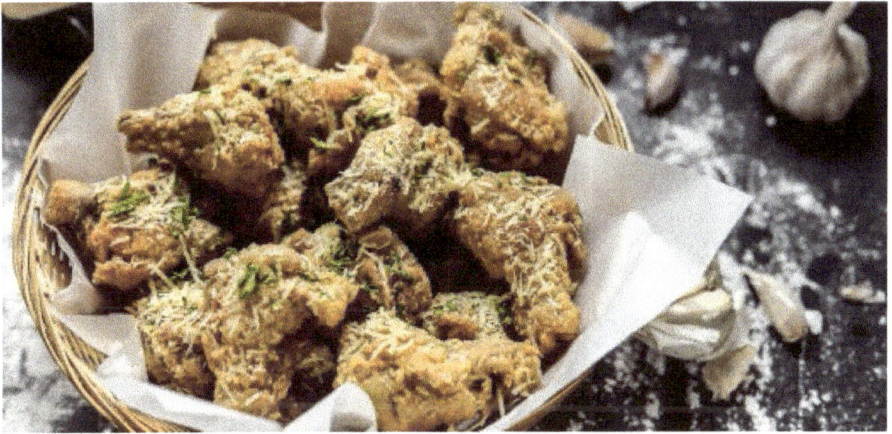

Pineapple & Ginger Chicken Kabobs

Prep Time:
20 minutes
Serve: 4

Ingredients:

- ¾ oz boneless and skinless chicken tenders
- ½ cup soy sauce
- ½ cup pineapple juice
- ¼ cup sesame oil
- 4 cloves garlic, chopped
- 1 tbsp fresh ginger, grated
- 4 scallions, chopped
- 2 tbsp toasted sesame seeds
- 1 A pinch of black pepper

Directions:

1.Skewer the chicken pieces into the skewers and trim any fat.

2.In a large sized bowl, mix the remaining ingredients.

3.Dip the skewered chicken into the seasoning bowl. Preheat your Air Fryer to 390 F.

4.Pat the chicken to dry using a towel and place in the Air Fryer cooking basket.

5.Cook for 5-7 minutes.

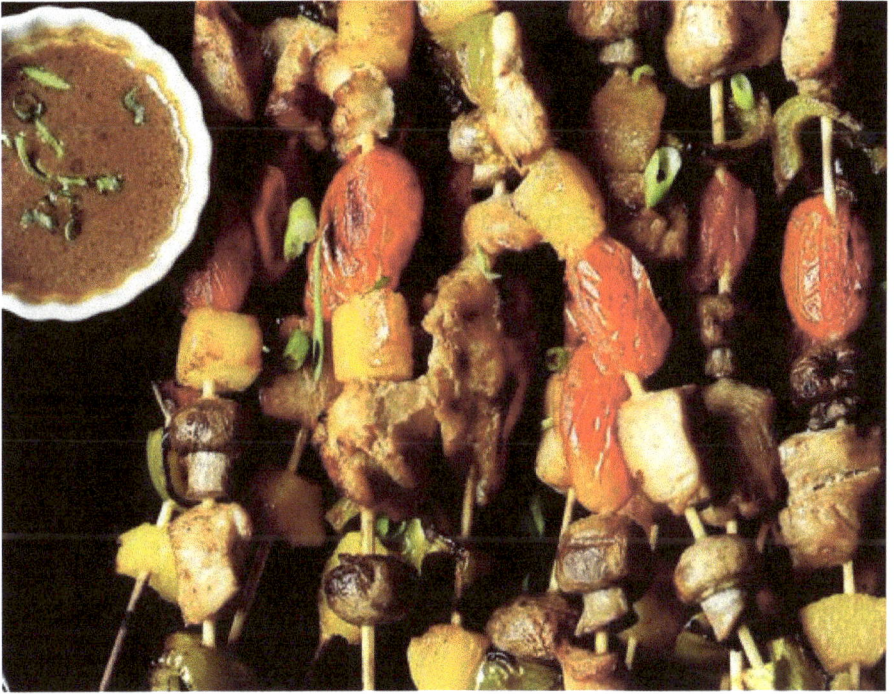

Worcestershire Chicken Breasts

Prep Time:
20 minutes
Serve: 6

Ingredients:

- ¼ cup flour
- ½ tbsp flour
- 5 chicken breasts, sliced
- 1 tbsp Worcestershire sauce
- 3 tbsp olive oil
- ¼ cup onions, chopped
- 1 ½ cups brown sugar
- ¼ cup yellow mustard
- ¾ cup water
- ½ cup ketchup

Directions:

1.Preheat your Fryer to 360 F. In a bowl, mix in flour, salt and pepper.

2.Cover the chicken slices with flour mixture and drizzle oil over the chicken.

3.In another bowl, mix brown sugar, water, ketchup, chopped onion, mustard, Worcestershire sauce and salt.

4.Transfer chicken to marinade mixture; set aside for 10 minutes.

5.Place the chicken in your Air Fryer's cooking basket and cook for 15 minutes.

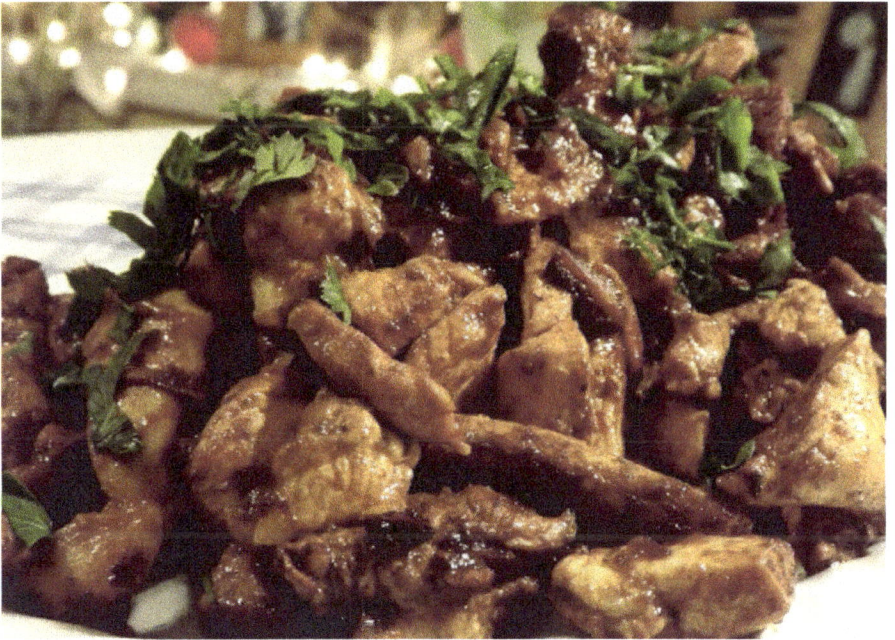

Sherry Grilled Chicken

Prep Time:
25 minutes
Serve: 2

Ingredients:

- 4 chicken breasts, cubed
- 2 garlic clove, minced
- ½ cup ketchup
- ½ tbsp ginger, minced
- ½ cup soy sauce
- 2 tbsp sherry
- ½ cup pineapple juice
- 2 tbsp apple cider vinegar
- ½ cup brown sugar

Directions:

1.Preheat your Air Fryer to 360 F. In a bowl, mix in ketchup, pineapple Juice, sugar, cider vinegar, ginger.

2.Heat the sauce in a frying pan over low heat. Cover chicken with the soy sauce and sherry; pour the hot sauce on top.

3.Set aside for 15 minutes to marinate. Place the chicken in the Air Fryer cooking basket and cook for 15 minutes.

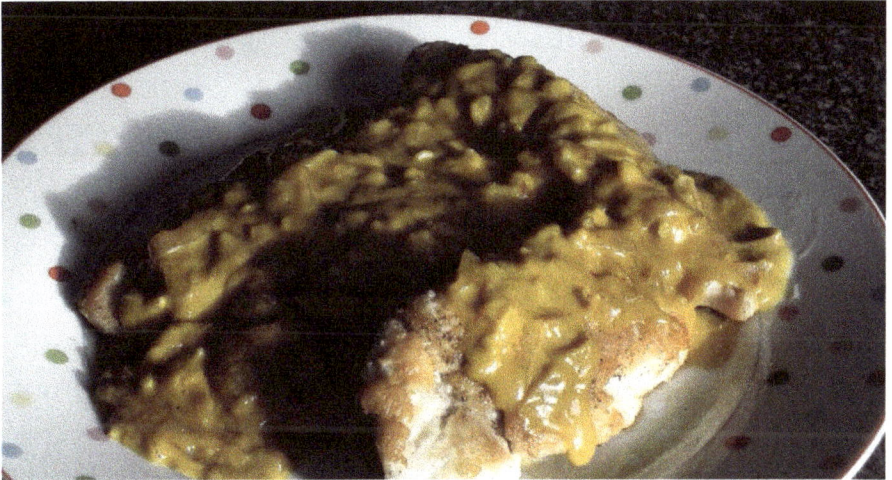

Mustard Chicken with Thyme

Prep Time:
20 minutes
Serve: 4

Ingredients:

- 4 garlic cloves, minced
- 8 chicken slices
- 1 tbsp thyme leaves
- ½ cup dry wine Salt as needed
- ½ cup Dijon mustard
- 2 cups breadcrumbs
- 2 tbsp melted butter
- 1 tbsp lemon zest
- 2 tbsp olive oil

Directions:

1.Preheat your Air Fryer to 350 F. In a bowl, mix garlic, salt, cloves, breadcrumbs, pepper, oil, butter and lemon zest.

2.In another bowl, mix mustard and wine.

3.Place chicken slices in the wine mixture and then in the crumb mixture.

4.Place the prepared chicken in the Air Fryer cooking basket and cook for 15 minutes.

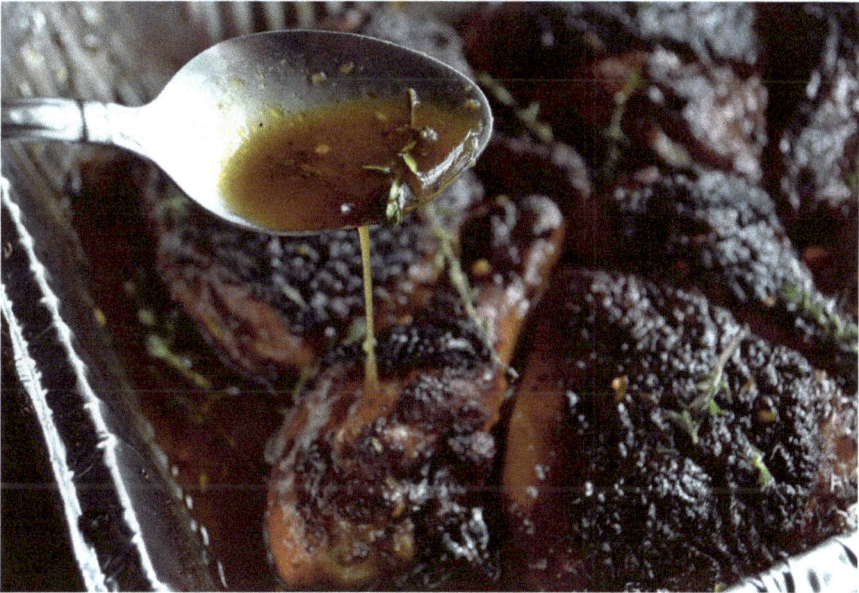

Shrimp Paste Chicken

Prep Time:
30 minutes
Serve: 2

Ingredients:

- 8 chicken wings, washed and cut into small portions
- ½ tbsp sugar
- 2 tbsp corn flour
- ½ tbsp wine
- 1 tbsp shrimp paste
- 1 tbsp ginger
- ½ tbsp olive oil

Directions:

1.Preheat your Air Fryer to 360 F. In a bowl, mix oil, ginger, wine and sugar.

2.Cover the chicken wings with the prepared marinade and top with flour.

3.Add the floured chicken to shrimp paste and coat it.

4.Place the prepared chicken in your Air Fryer's cooking basket and cook for 20 minutes, until crispy on the outside.

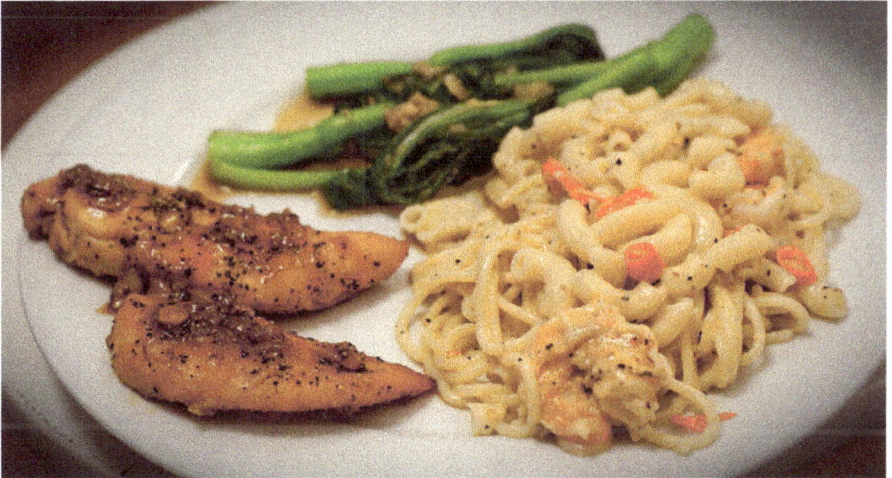

Beef and Zucchinis Bowls

Prep Time:
10 minutes
Cook Time:
8 hours
Serve: 4

Ingredients:

- 1 pound beef loin, cut into strips
- 1 tablespoon olive oil
- ¼ cup beef stock
- ½ teaspoon sweet paprika
- ½ teaspoon chili powder
- 2 small zucchinis, cubed
- 1 tablespoon balsamic vinegar
- 1 tablespoon chives, chopped

Directions:

1.In your slow cooker, mix the beef with the oil, stock, and the other ingredients, toss, put the lid on and cook on Low for 8 hours.

2.Divide the mix between plates and serve.

Nutrition: 250 calories,31.1g protein, 2.4g carbohydrates, 13.2g fat, 0.9g fiber, 81mg cholesterol, 121mg sodium, 566mg potassium.

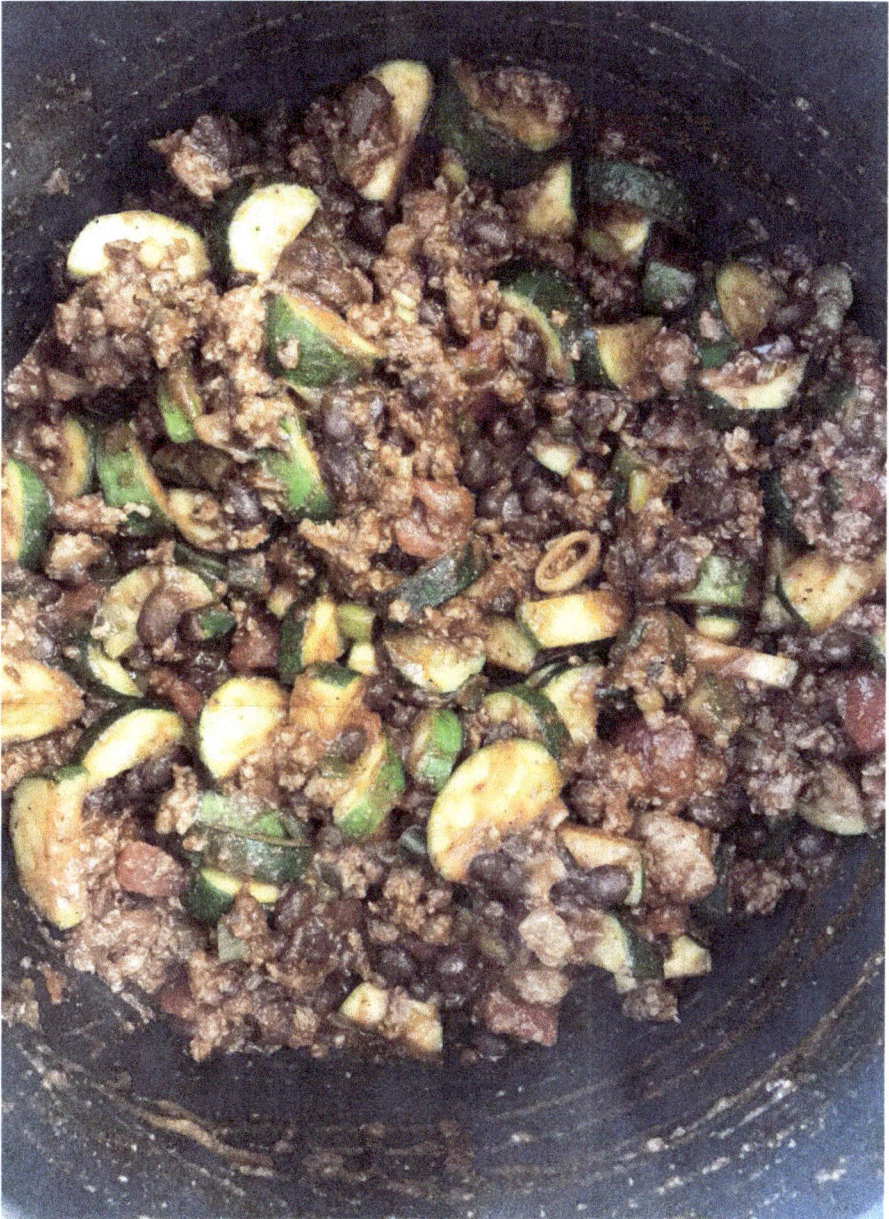

Onion Beef with Olives

Prep Time:
10 minutes
Cook Time:
8 hours
Serve: 4

Ingredients:

- 1 pound beef tenderloin, sliced
- ½ cup tomato passata
- 1 red onion, sliced
- 1 cup kalamata olives, pitted and halved
- Juice of ½ lime
- ¼ cup beef stock
- 1 tablespoon chives, hopped

Directions:

1. In your slow cooker, mix the beef slices with the passata, onion, olives, and the other ingredients, toss, put the lid on and cook on Low for 8 hours.

2. Divide the mix between plates and serve.

Nutrition: 288 calories,33.8g protein, 5.5g carbohydrates, 14g fat, 1.7g fiber, 104mg cholesterol, 410mg sodium, 458mg potassium.

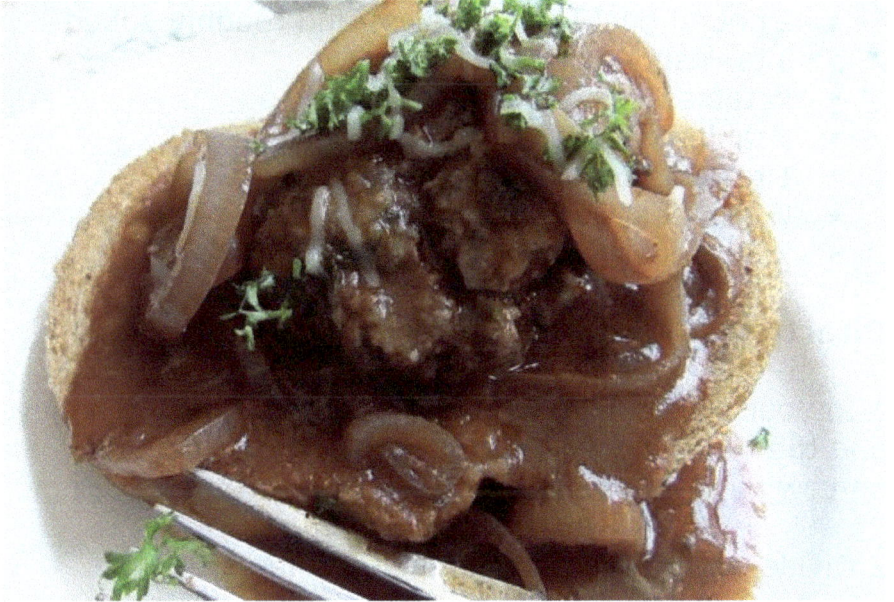

Beef Mix

Prep Time:
10 minutes
Cook Time:
8 hours
Serve: 4

Ingredients:

- 1 pound beef loin, boneless and roughly cubed
- 3 tablespoons honey
- ½ tablespoons oregano, dried
- 1 tablespoon garlic, minced
- 1 tablespoon olive oil
- ½ cup beef stock
- ½ teaspoon sweet paprika

Directions:

1.In your slow cooker, mix the beef loin with the honey, and the other ingredients, toss, put the lid on and cook on Low for 8 hours.

2.Divide everything between plates and serve.

Nutrition: 292 calories,31g protein, 14.2g carbohydrates, 13.1g fat, 0.4g fiber, 81mg cholesterol, 161mg sodium, 434mg potassium.

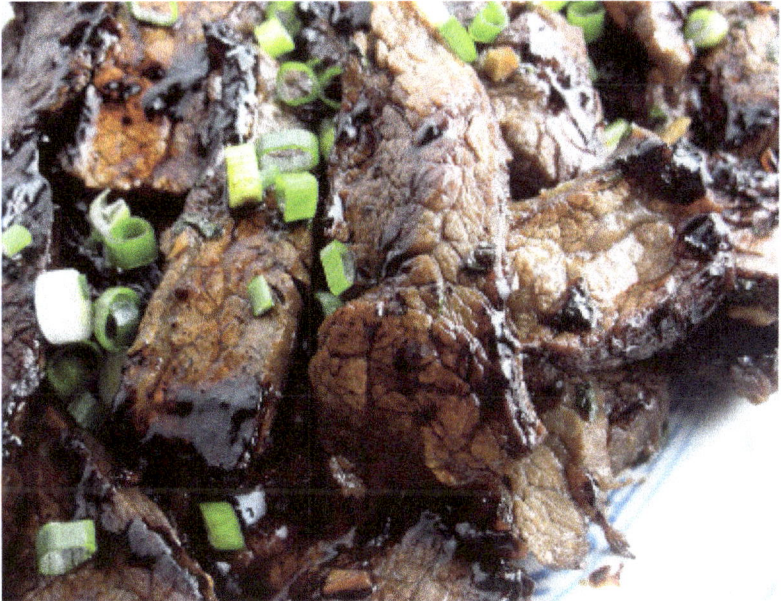

Beef with Yogurt Sauce

Prep Time:
10 minutes
Cook Time:
8 hours
Serve: 4

Ingredients:

- 1 pound beef loin, cubed
- 1 teaspoon garam masala
- ½ teaspoon turmeric powder
- 1 cup beef stock
- 1 teaspoon garlic, minced
- ½ cup Greek-style yogurt
- 1 tablespoon chives, chopped

Directions:

1.In your slow cooker, mix the beef with the turmeric, garam masala, and the other ingredients, toss, put the lid on and cook on Low for 8 hours.

2.Divide everything into bowls and serve.

Nutrition: 228 calories,33.8g protein, 1.5g carbohydrates, 9.6g fat, 0.1g fiber, 82mg cholesterol, 269mg sodium, 469mg potassium.

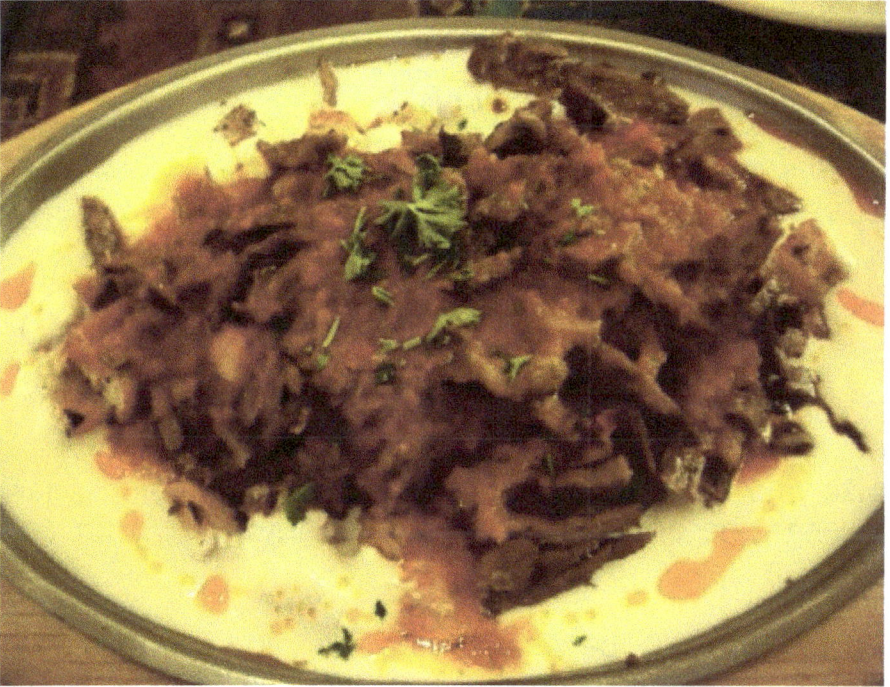

Beans Mix with Meat

Prep Time:
10 minutes
Cook Time:
8 hours
Serve: 4

Ingredients:

- 1 red bell pepper, chopped
- 1 pound beef loin, cubed
- 1 tablespoon olive oil
- 1 cup canned black beans, drained and rinsed
- ½ cup tomato sauce
- 1 yellow onion, chopped
- 1 teaspoon Italian seasoning
- 1 tablespoon oregano, chopped

Directions:

1.In your slow cooker, mix the beef with the bell pepper, oil, and the other ingredients, toss, put the lid on and cook on Low for 8 hours.

2.Divide the mix between plates and serve.

Nutrition: 437 calories,41.9g protein, 37.6g carbohydrates, 14.3g fat, 9.3g fiber, 81mg cholesterol, 228mg sodium, 1322mg potassium.

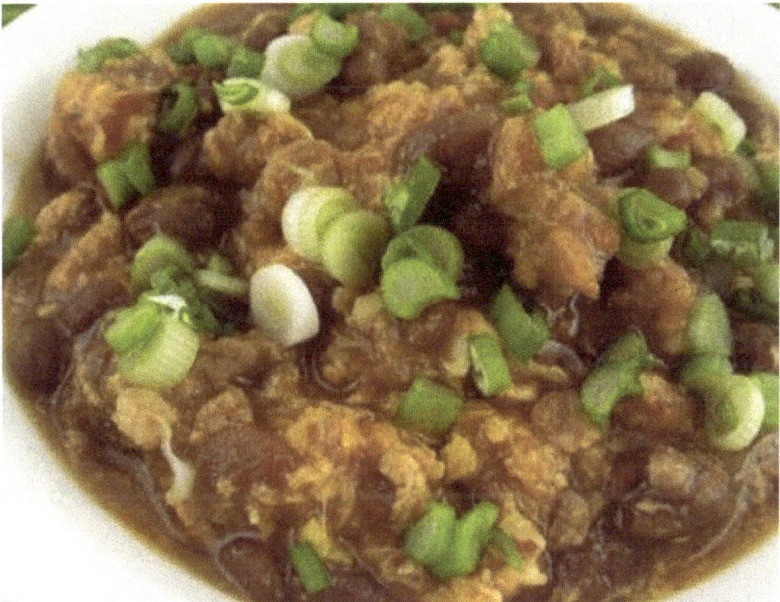

Beef and Spinach Bowls

Prep Time:
10 minutes
Cook Time:
7 hours
Serve: 4

Ingredients:

- 1 red onion, sliced
- 1-pound beef loin, cubed
- 1 cup tomato passata
- 1 cup baby spinach
- 1 teaspoon olive oil
- ½ cup beef stock
- 1 tablespoon basil, chopped

Directions:

1.In your slow cooker, mix the beef with the onion, passata, and the other ingredients except for the spinach, toss, put the lid on and cook on Low for 6 hours and 30 minutes.

2.Add the spinach, toss, put the lid on, cook on Low for 30 minutes more, divide into bowls, and serve.

Nutrition: 246 calories,31.7g protein, 4.5g carbohydrates, 11.1g fat, 0.8g fiber, 81mg cholesterol, 94mg sodium, 470mg potassium.

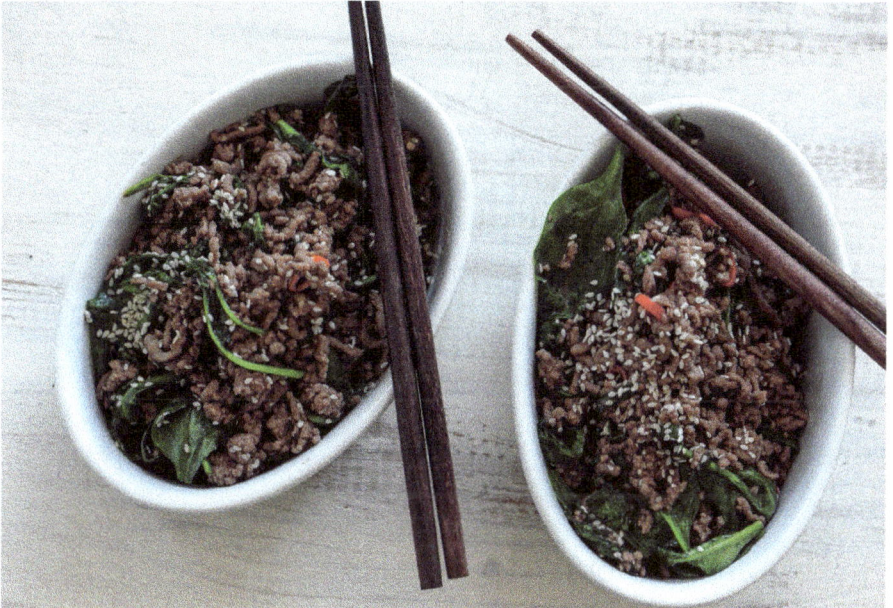

Chilies Meat Mix

Prep Time:
10 minutes
Cook Time:
7 hours
Serve: 4

Ingredients:

- 1 pound beef loin, cubed
- 1 tablespoon olive oil
- ½ green bell pepper, chopped
- 1 red onion, sliced
- ½ red bell pepper, chopped
- 1 garlic clove, minced
- 2 ounces canned green chilies, chopped
- ½ cup tomato passata
- 1 tablespoon chili powder
- 1 tablespoon cilantro, chopped

Directions:

1.In your slow cooker, mix the beef with the oil, bell pepper, and the other ingredients, toss, put the lid on and cook on Low for 7 hours.

2.Divide into bowls and serve right away.

Nutrition: 263 calories,31.3g protein, 5.9g carbohydrates, 13.4g fat, 1.5g fiber, 81mg cholesterol, 83mg sodium, 494mg potassium.

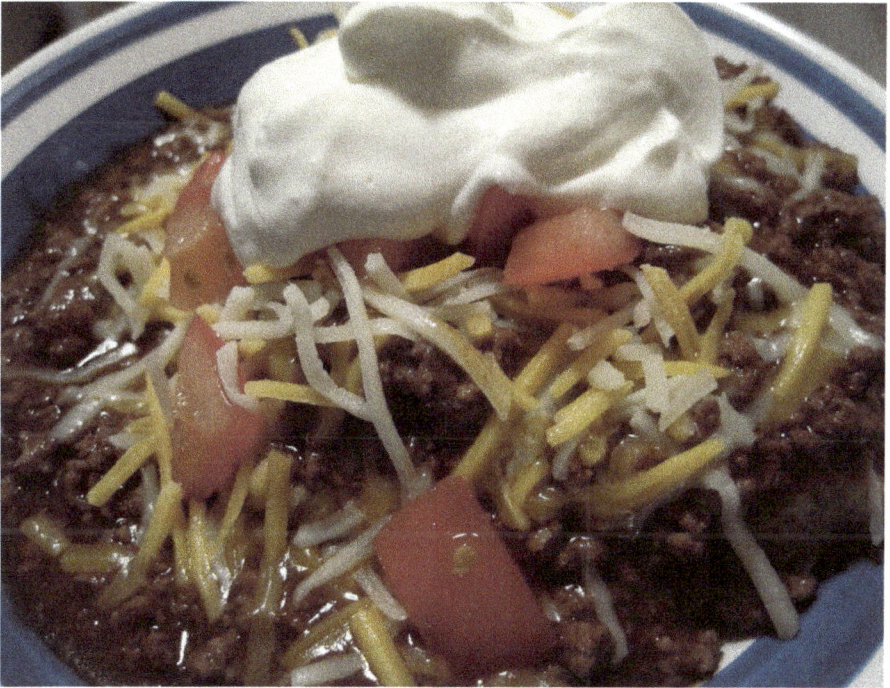

Fragrant Tenderloin

Prep Time:
10 minutes
Cook Time:
8 hours
Serve: 2

Ingredients:

- 2 beef tenderloin
- ½ cup tomato juice, fresh
- 1 tablespoon balsamic vinegar
- 1 tablespoon mustard
- 1 tablespoon chives, chopped

Directions:

1.In your slow cooker, combine the meat with the tomato juice, and the other ingredients, toss, put the lid on, and cook on Low for 8 hours.

2.Divide between plates and serve with a side salad.

Nutrition: 214 calories,26.5g protein, 4.7g carbohydrates, 9.4g fat, 1.1g fiber, 78mg cholesterol, 214mg sodium, 491mg potassium.

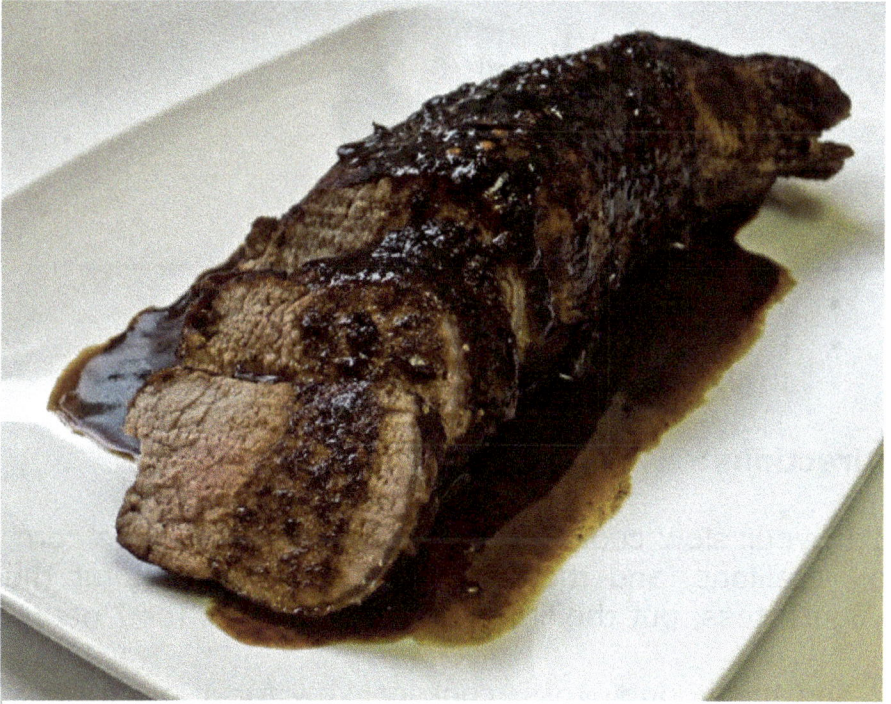

Meat and Corn Mix

Prep Time:
10 minutes
Cook Time:
8 hours
Serve: 2

Ingredients:

- 2 teaspoons olive oil
- 3 scallions, chopped
- 1 pound beef loin, cubed
- 1 cup of corn kernels
- ½ cup Greek-style yogurt
- ½ cup beef stock
- 2 garlic cloves, minced
- 1 tablespoon pomegranate sauce
- 1 tablespoon parsley, chopped

Directions:

1.In your slow cooker, combine the beef with the corn, oil, scallions, and the other ingredients except for the yogurt, toss, put the lid on and cook on Low for 7 hours.

2.Add the yogurt, toss, cook on Low for 1 more hour, divide into bowls and serve.

Nutrition: 284 calories,32.8g protein, 10.2g carbohydrates, 13.3g fat, 1.5g fiber, 81mg cholesterol, 174mg sodium, 548mg potassium.

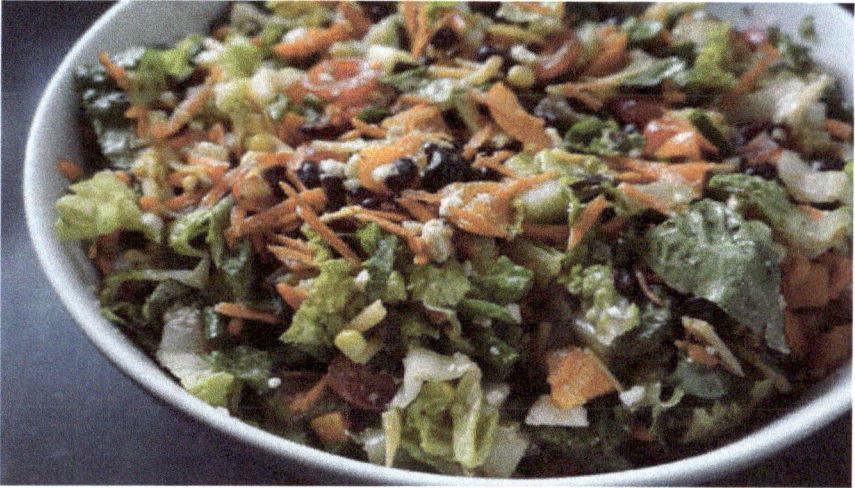

Lime Beef Mix

Prep Time:
10 minutes
Cook Time:
8 hours
 Serve: 4

Ingredients:

- 1 pound beef loin, cubed
- 1 tablespoon olive oil
- 3 garlic cloves, minced
- ½ yellow onion, chopped
- ½ cup beef stock
- 1 tablespoon apple cider vinegar
- 1 tablespoon lime zest, grated

Directions:

1.In your slow cooker, mix the beef with the oil, garlic, and the other ingredients, toss, put the lid on, and cook on Low for 8 hours.

2.Divide everything between plates and serve.

Nutrition: 249 calories,31g protein, 2.3g carbohydrates, 13.1g fat, 0.5g fiber, 81mg cholesterol, 161mg sodium, 436mg potassium.

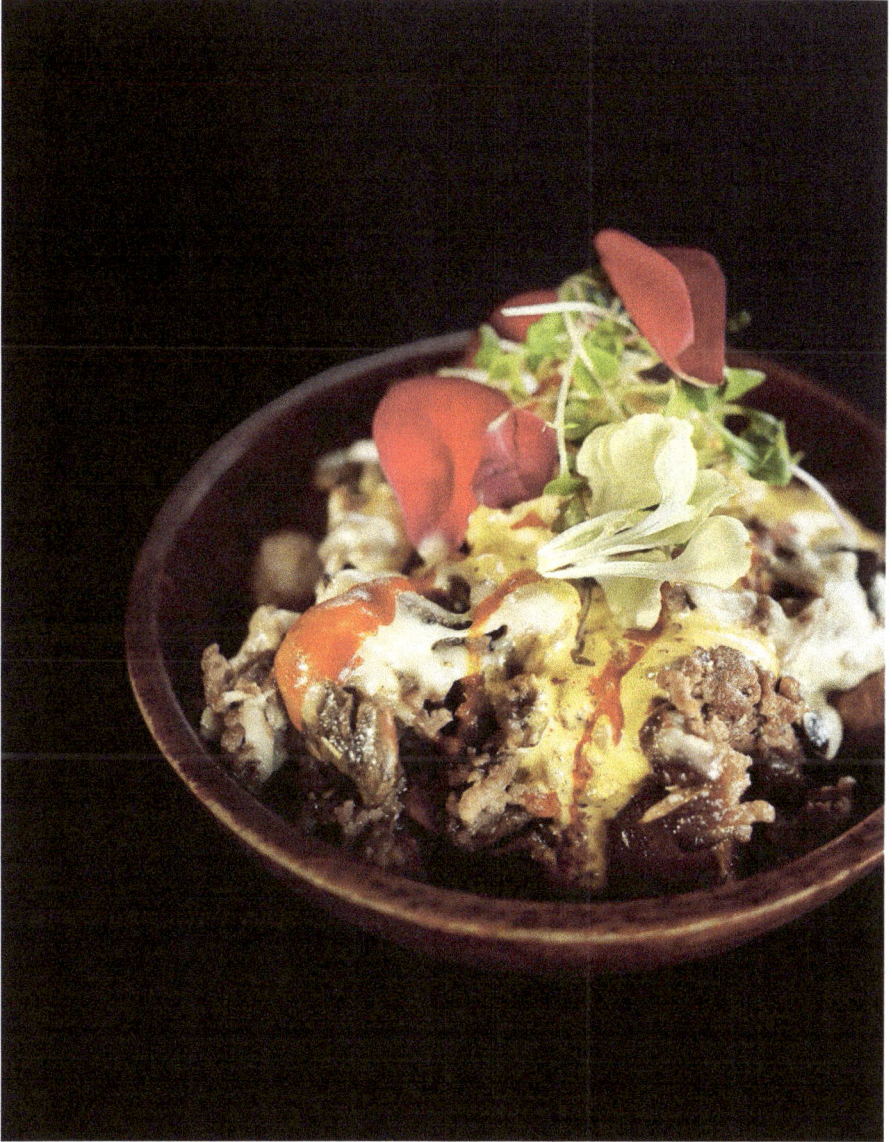

Coriander Beef Chops

Prep Time:
10 minutes
Cook Time:
6 hours
Serve: 4

Ingredients:

- ½ pound beef chops
- ¼ tablespoons olive oil
- 2 garlic clove, minced
- ¼ teaspoon chili powder
- ½ cup beef stock
- ½ teaspoon coriander, ground
- ¼ teaspoon mustard powder
- 1 tablespoon tarragon, chopped

Directions:

1.Grease your slow cooker with the oil and mix the beef chops with the garlic, stock, and the other ingredients inside.

2.Toss, put the lid on, cook on Low for 6 hours, divide between plates and serve with a side salad.

Nutrition: 204 calories,11.5g protein, 1.6g carbohydrates, 16.3g fat, 0.1g fiber, 44mg cholesterol, 456mg sodium, 41mg potassium.

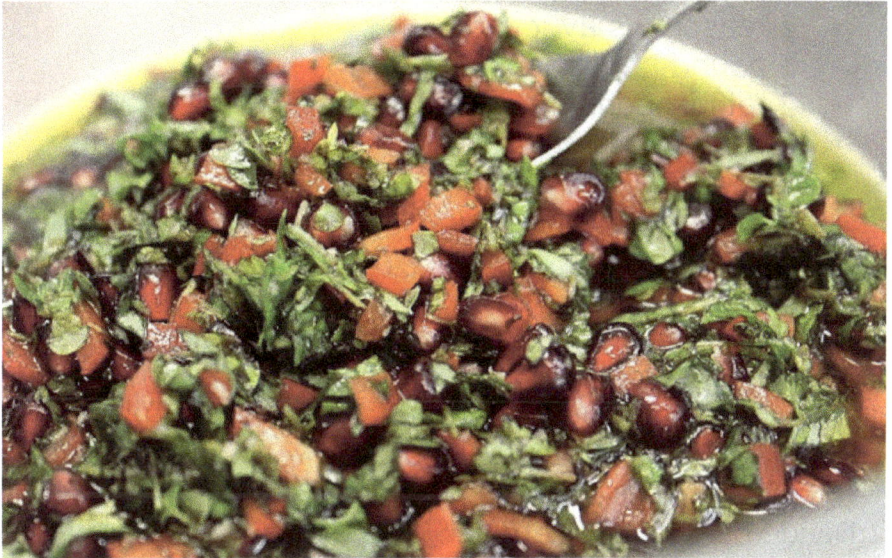

Spicy Lime Beef Chops

Prep Time:
10 minutes
Cook Time:
5 hours
Serve: 4

Ingredients:

- 2 teaspoons avocado oil
- 1 pound beef chops, bone-in
- 2 tablespoons mayonnaise, low-fat
- ½ tablespoon honey
- ¼ cup beef stock
- ½ tablespoon lime juice

Directions:

1.In your slow cooker, mix the beef chops with the oil, honey, and the other ingredients, toss well, put the lid on, and cook on High for 5 hours.

2.Divide beef chops between plates and serve.

Nutrition: 253 calories,34.7g protein, 4.6g carbohydrates, 9.9g fat, 0.1g fiber, 103mg cholesterol, 177mg sodium, 480mg potassium.

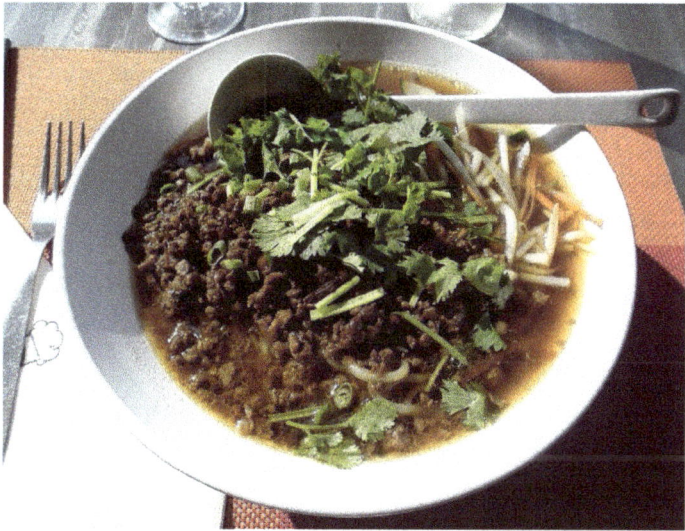

Chives Turmeric Beef

Prep Time:
 10 minutes
Cook Time:
5 hours
Serve: 4

Ingredients:

- 1 pound beef chops
- 2 teaspoons avocado oil
- 1 teaspoon turmeric powder
- ½ teaspoon sweet paprika
- 1 cup beef stock
- 1 red onion, sliced
- 1 tablespoon chives, chopped

Directions:

1.In your slow cooker, mix the beef chops with the oil, turmeric, and the other ingredients, toss, put the lid on and cook on High for 5 hours.

2.Divide everything between plates and serve.

Nutrition: 486 calories,38.8g protein, 15.5g carbohydrates, 29.6g fat, 3g fiber, 54mg cholesterol, 204mg sodium, 779mg potassium.

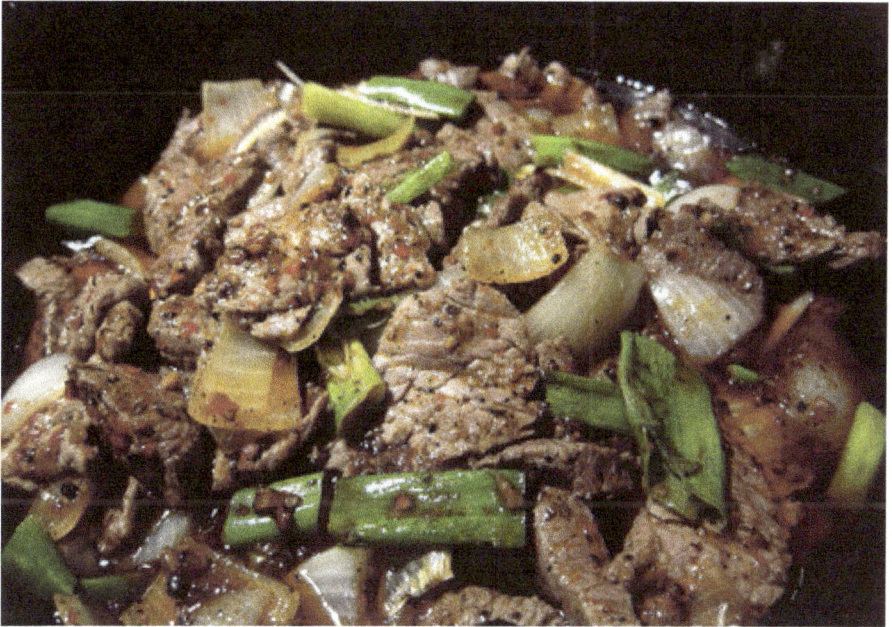

Chili and Garlic Beef

Prep Time:
10 minutes
Cook Time:
4 hours
Serve: 4

Ingredients:

- 1 pound beef chops
- 2 teaspoons avocado oil
- 2 scallions, chopped
- 1 green chili pepper, minced
- ½ teaspoon turmeric powder
- 1 teaspoon chili powder
- ½ cup vegetable stock
- 2 garlic cloves, minced

Directions:

1.In your slow cooker, mix the beef chops with the oil, scallions, and the other ingredients, toss, put the lid on and cook on High for 4 hours.

2.Divide everything between plates and serve.

Nutrition: 310 calories,23.3g protein, 2.8g carbohydrates, 21.8g fat, 0.9g fiber, 60mg cholesterol, 470mg sodium, 89mg potassium.

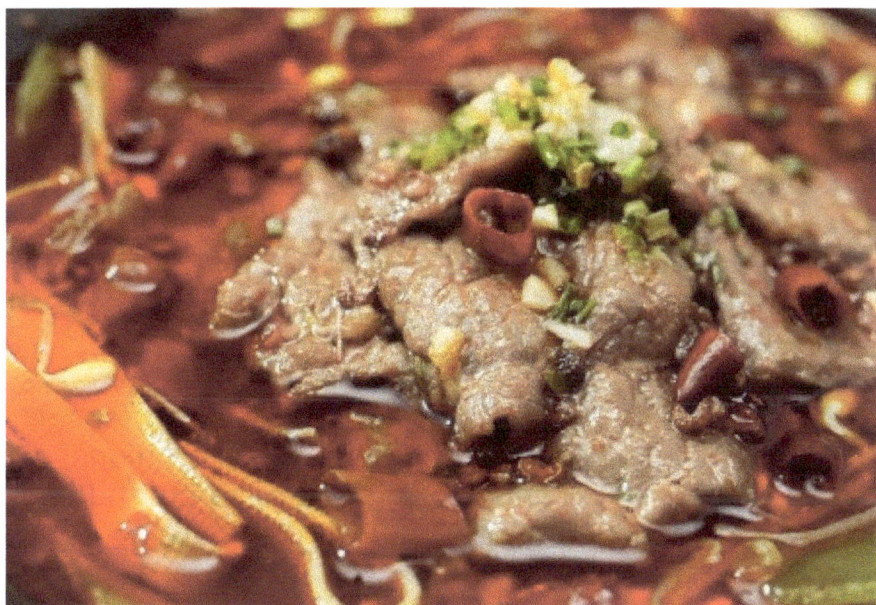

Beef Mix with Onions

Prep Time:
10 minutes
Cook Time:
7 hours
Serve: 4

Ingredients:

- 1 pound beef loin, cubed
- 2 teaspoons olive oil
- 2 red onions, sliced
- 1 cup Greek-style yogurt
- ¼ cup beef stock
- 1 teaspoon chili powder
- ½ teaspoon rosemary, dried
- 1 tablespoon parsley, chopped

Directions:

1.In your slow cooker, mix the beef with the onions, oil, and the other ingredients, toss, put the lid on and cook on low for 7 hours.

2.Divide everything between plates and serve.

Nutrition: 252 calories,31.2g protein, 5.7g carbohydrates, 12g fat, 1.5g fiber, 81mg cholesterol, 121mg sodium, 493mg potassium.

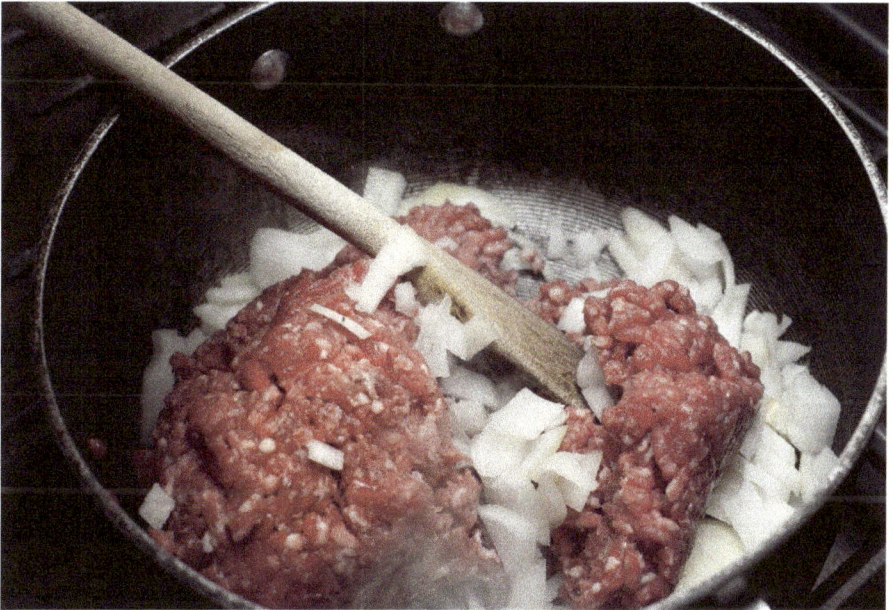

Beef and Okra Saute

Prep Time:
10 minutes
Cook Time:
6 hours
Serve: 4

Ingredients:

- 1 pound beef loin, cubed
- 1 cup okra, sliced
- 2 teaspoons olive oil
- 1 red onion, chopped
- ¼ cup beef stock
- ½ teaspoon chili powder
- ½ teaspoon turmeric powder
- 1 cup tomato passata

Directions:

1.In your slow cooker, combine the beef with the okra, oil, and the other ingredients, toss, put the lid on and cook on High for 6 hours.

2.Divide the mix between plates and serve.

Nutrition: 258 calories,31.7g protein, 6.4g carbohydrates, 12g fat, 1.6g fiber, 81mg cholesterol, 118mg sodium, 522mg potassium.

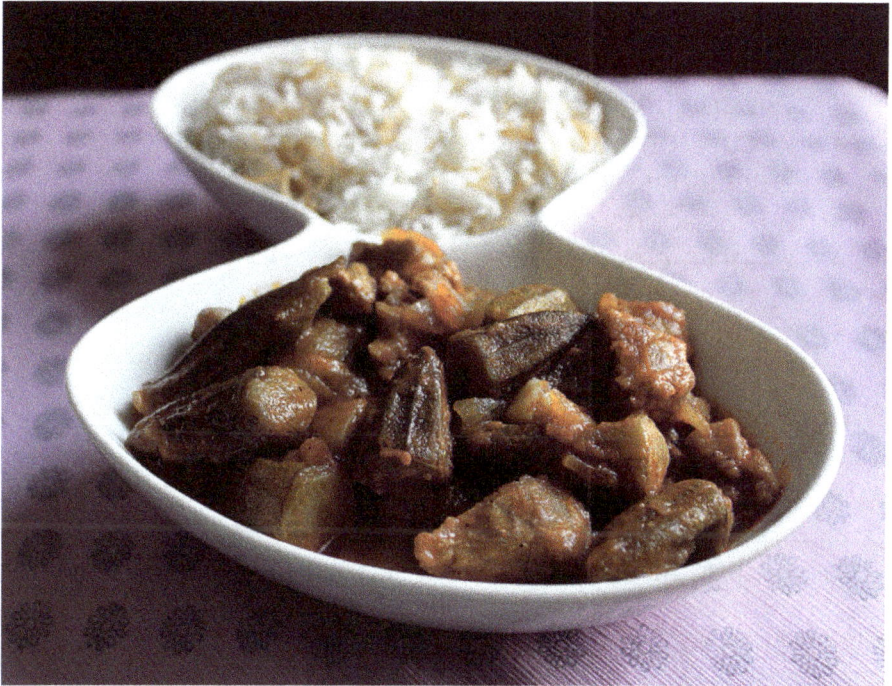

Chives Beef with Cumin

Prep Time:
10 minutes
Cook Time:
4 hours
Serve: 4

Ingredients:

- 1 pound beef chops
- ½ cup chives, chopped
- ½ cup tomato passata
- 2 scallions, chopped
- 2 teaspoons olive oil
- 2 garlic cloves, minced
- ½ teaspoon sweet paprika
- 1 teaspoon cumin, ground

Directions:

1.In your slow cooker, mix the beef chops with the chives, passata, and the other ingredients, toss, put the lid on and cook on High for 4 hours,

2.Divide the mix between plates and serve.

Nutrition: 334 calories,22.8g protein, 2.5g carbohydrates, 25.6g fat, 0.5g fiber, 85mg cholesterol, 58mg sodium, 60mg potassium.

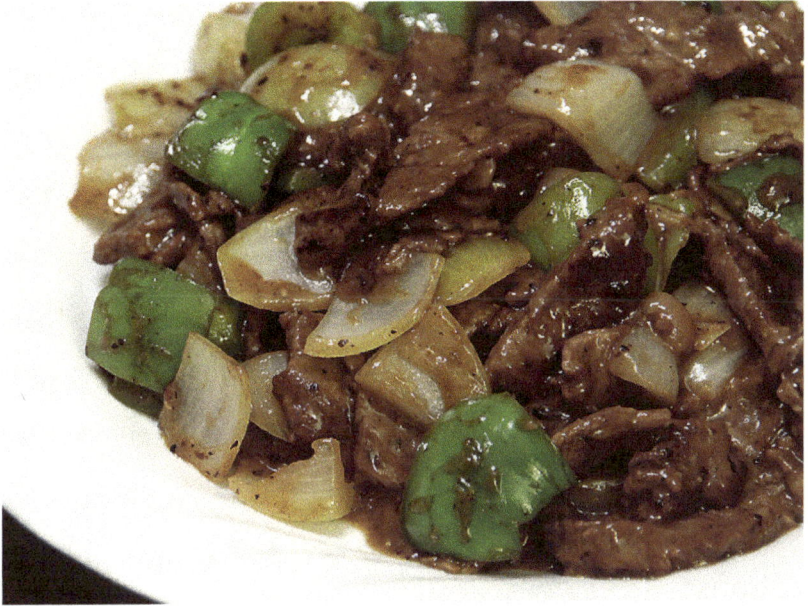

Oregano Beef with Tomato Sauce

Prep Time:
10 minutes
Cook Time:
4 hours
Serve: 4

Ingredients:

- 1 pound beef loin, cubed
- 1 tablespoon olive oil
- 1 tablespoon balsamic vinegar
- ½ tablespoon lemon juice
- 1 tablespoon oregano, chopped
- ½ cup tomato sauce
- 1 red onion, chopped
- ½ teaspoon chili powder

Directions:

1.In your slow cooker, mix the beef with the oil, vinegar, lemon juice, and the other ingredients, toss, put the lid on and cook on High for 4 hours.

2.Divide the mix between plates and serve right away.

Nutrition: 260 calories,31.2g protein, 5.2g carbohydrates, 13.3g fat, 1.7g fiber, 81mg cholesterol, 228mg sodium, 557mg potassium.

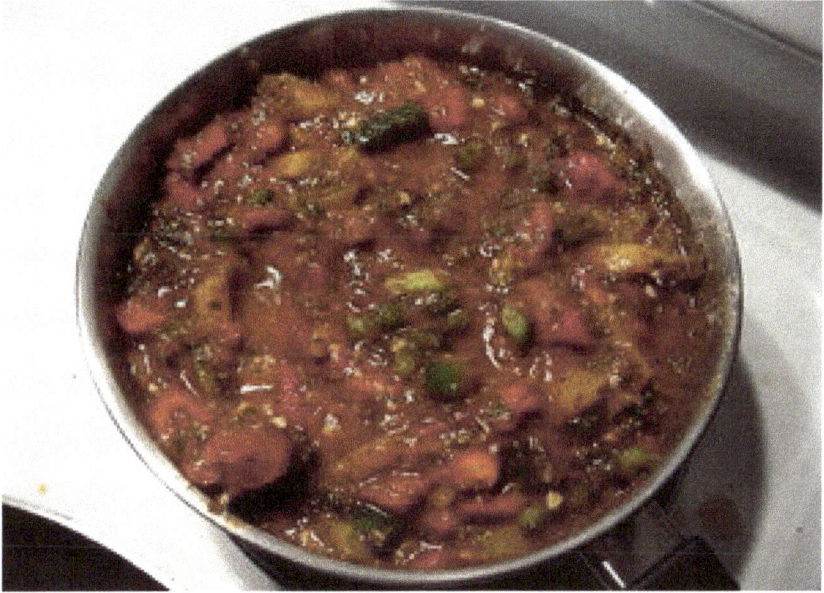

Beef and Green Beans Bowls

Prep Time:
10 minutes
Cook Time:
6 hours
Serve: 4

Ingredients:

- 1 pound beef loin, cubed
- 1 tablespoon balsamic vinegar
- 1 cup green beans, trimmed and halved
- 1 tablespoon lime juice
- 1 tablespoon avocado oil
- ½ teaspoon rosemary, dried
- 1 cup beef stock
- 1 tablespoon chives, chopped

Directions:

1.In your slow cooker, mix the beef loin with the green beans, vinegar, and the other ingredients, toss, put the lid on, and cook on Low for 6 hours.

2.Divide the mix between plates and serve.

Nutrition: 225 calories,31.6g protein, 2.3g carbohydrates, 10.1g fat, 1.2g fiber, 81mg cholesterol, 230mg sodium, 493mg potassium.

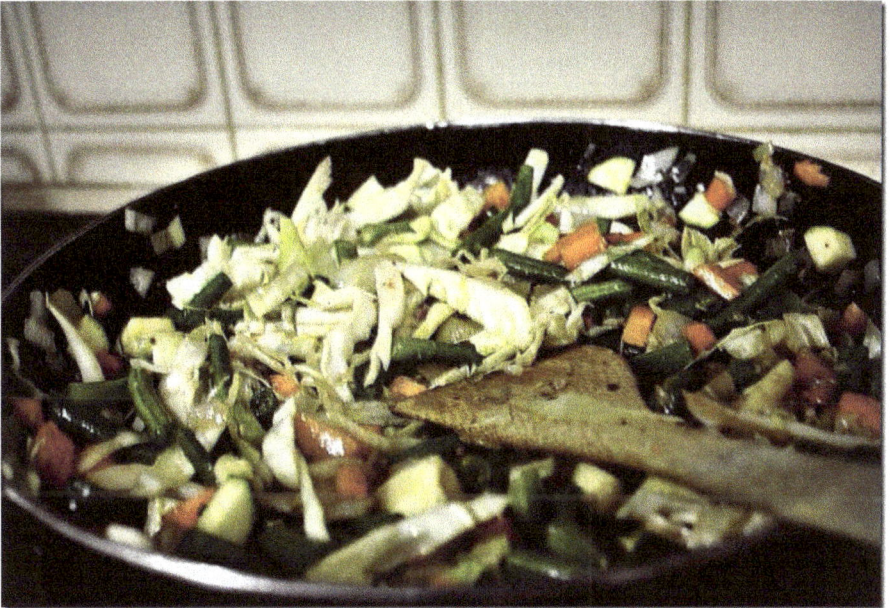

Mint Meat Chops

Prep Time:
10 minutes
Cook Time:
4 hours
Serve: 5

Ingredients:

- 2 tablespoons olive oil
- 1 pound beef chops
- 1 tablespoon mint, chopped
- ½ teaspoon garam masala
- ½ cup coconut cream
- 1 red onion, chopped
- 2 tablespoons garlic, minced

Directions:

1.In your slow cooker, mix the beef chops with the oil, mint, and the other ingredients, toss, put the lid on and cook on High for 4 hours.

2.Divide the mix between plates and serve warm.

Nutrition: 360 calories,19g protein, 4.6g carbohydrates, 29.9g fat, 1.2g fiber, 68mg cholesterol, 128mg sodium, 127mg potassium.

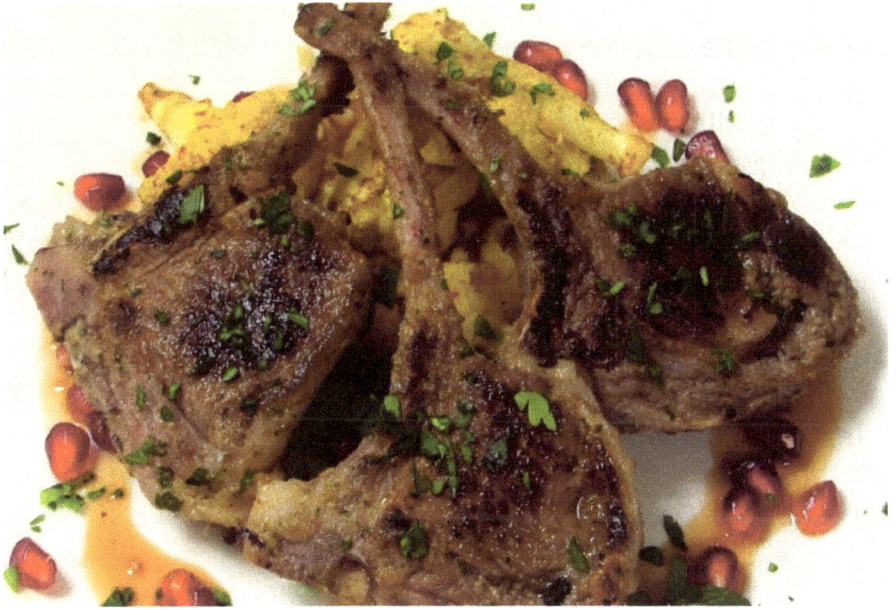

Beef and Vegetable Plates

Prep Time:
10 minutes
Cook Time:
7 hours
Serve: 4

Ingredients:

- 1 tablespoon avocado oil
- 1 pound beef loin, cubed
- 2 scallions, chopped
- 1 cup artichoke hearts
- ½ teaspoon chili powder
- 1 cup tomato passata
- ¼ tablespoon dill, chopped

Directions:

1.In your slow cooker, combine the beef with the artichokes and the other ingredients, toss, put the lid on and cook on Low for 7 hours.

2.Divide the mix between plates and serve.

Nutrition: 230 calories,31.2g protein, 4.4g carbohydrates, 10g fat, 1g fiber, 81mg cholesterol, 167mg sodium, 430mg potassium.

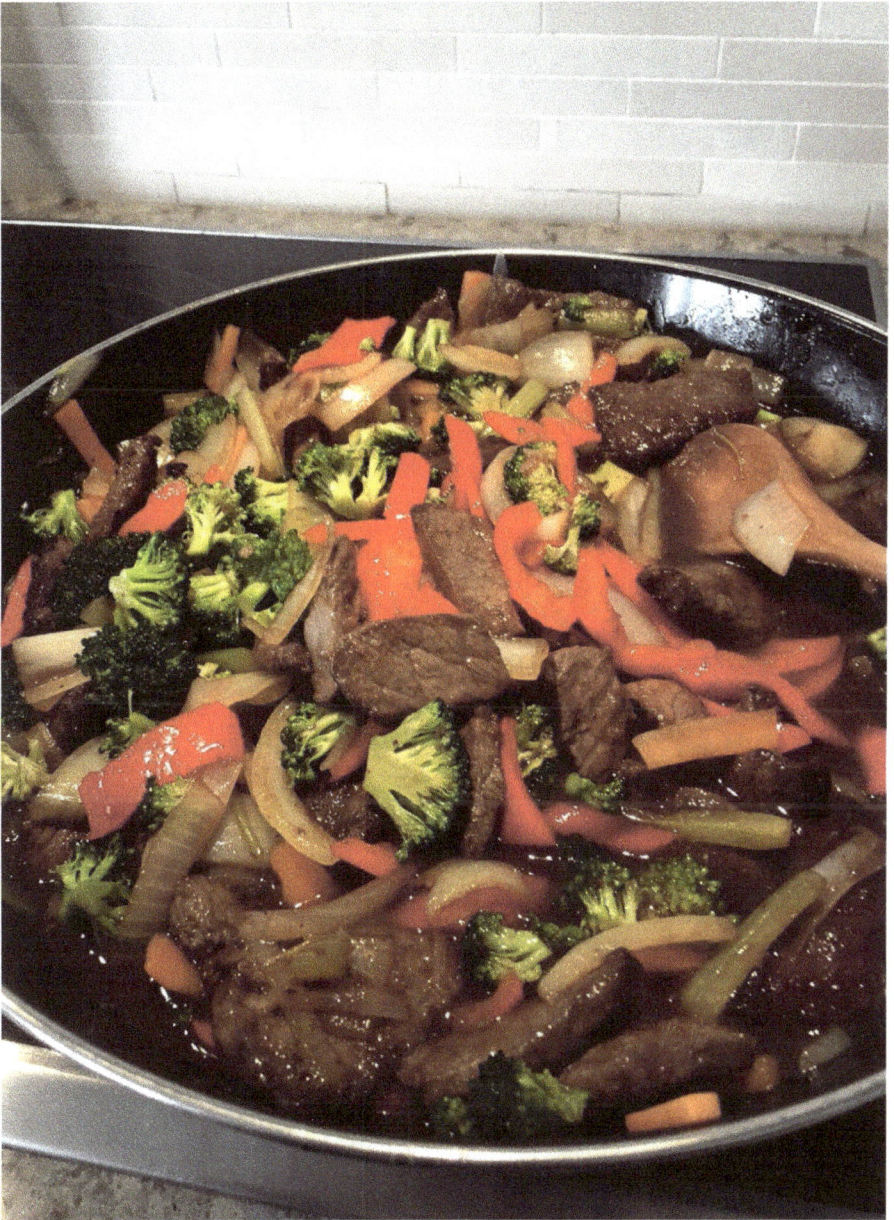

Beef with Paprika and Sweet Potato

Prep Time:
10 minutes
Cook Time:
4 hours
Serve: 4

Ingredients:

- 1 pound beef loin, roughly cubed
- 2 sweet potatoes, peeled and cubed
- ½ cup beef stock
- ½ cup tomato sauce
- ½ teaspoon sweet paprika
- ½ teaspoon coriander, ground
- 1 tablespoon avocado oil
- 1 tablespoon balsamic vinegar
- 1 tablespoon cilantro, chopped

Directions:

1.In your slow cooker, mix the beef with the potatoes, stock, sauce, and the other ingredients toss, put the lid on and cook on High for 4 hours

2.Divide everything between plates and serve.

Nutrition: 266 calories,31.7g protein, 12.5g carbohydrates, 10.1g fat, 2.3g fiber, 81mg cholesterol, 324mg sodium, 829mg potassium.

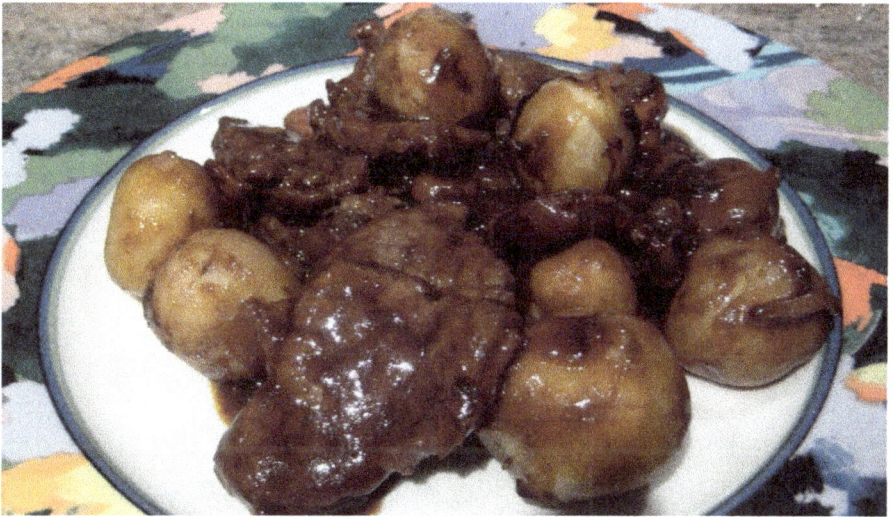

Oregano and Basil Beef

Prep Time:
10 minutes
Cook Time:
4 hours
Serve: 4

Ingredients:

- 1 teaspoon olive oil
- 1 pound beef loin, cubed
- 1 cup cherry tomatoes, halved
- 1 tablespoon basil, chopped
- ½ teaspoon rosemary, dried
- 1 tablespoon oregano, chopped
- 1 cup beef stock
- ½ teaspoon sweet paprika
- 1 tablespoon parsley, chopped

Directions:

1.Grease the slow cooker with the oil and mix the beef with the tomatoes, basil, and the other ingredients inside.

2.Toss, put the lid on, cook on High for 4 hours, divide the mix between plates and serve.

Nutrition: 234 calories,31.6g protein, 2.8g carbohydrates, 11g fat, 1.2g fiber, 81mg cholesterol, 261mg sodium, 558mg potassium.

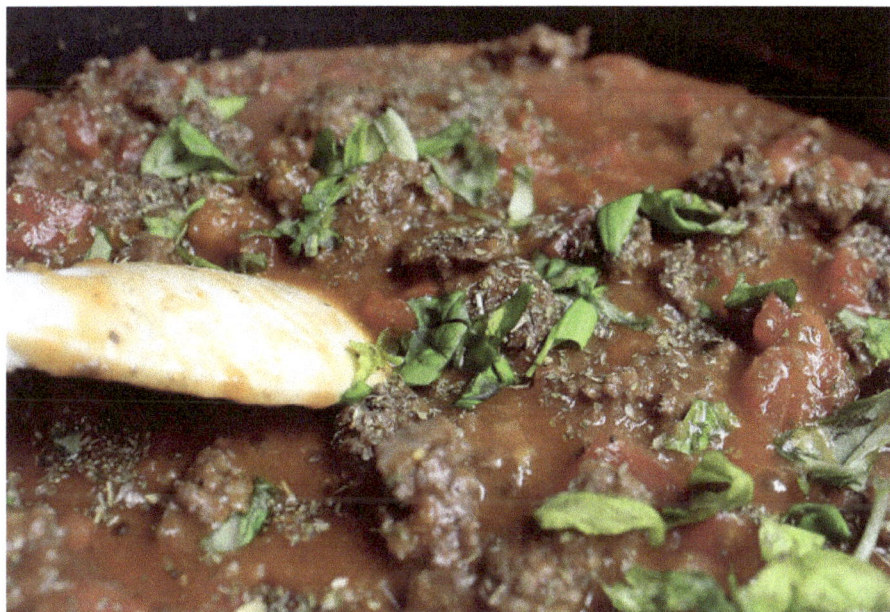

Tender Beef with Eggplants

Prep Time:
10 minutes
Cook Time:
7 hours
Serve: 4

Ingredients:

- 1 pound beef loin, cubed
- 1 eggplant, cubed
- 2 scallions, chopped
- 2 garlic cloves, minced
- ½ cup beef stock
- ¼ cup tomato sauce
- 1 teaspoon sweet paprika
- 1 tablespoon chives, chopped

Directions:

1.In your slow cooker, mix the beef loin with the scallions, eggplant, and the other ingredients, toss, put the lid on and cook on Low for 7 hours.

2.Divide the mix between plates and serve right away.

Nutrition: 247 calories,32.3g protein, 8.9g carbohydrates, 9.9g fat, 4.7g fiber, 81mg cholesterol, 244mg sodium, 756mg potassium.

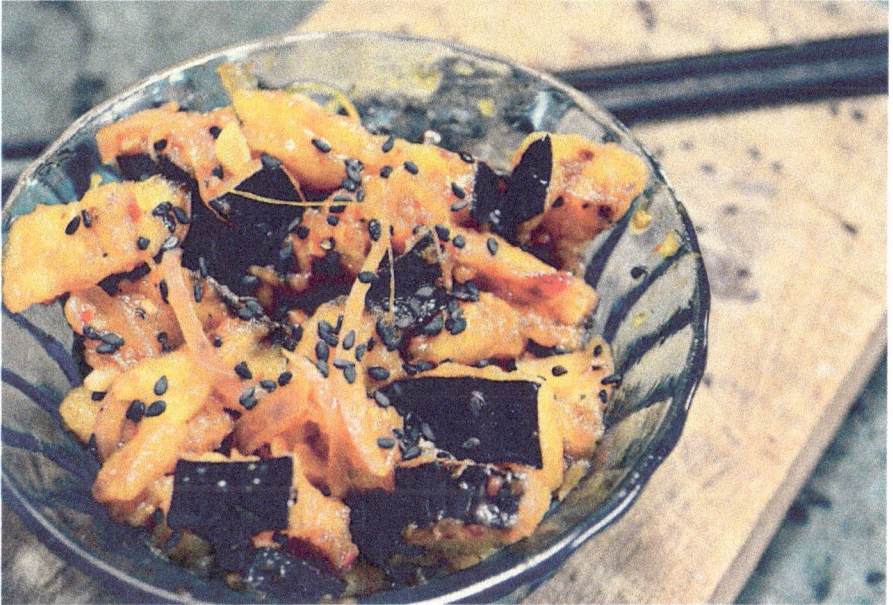

Lemon Beef with Onions

Prep Time:
10 minutes
Cook Time:
7 hours
Serve: 4

Ingredients:

- 1 pound beef loin, cubed
- 1 red onion, sliced
- ½ cup tomato sauce
- 1 tablespoon balsamic vinegar
- 1 tablespoon lemon juice
- 1 tablespoon lemon zest, grated
- 1 teaspoon olive oil
- 3 garlic cloves, chopped
- 1 tablespoon chives, chopped

Directions:

1.In your slow cooker, mix the beef with the onion, tomato sauce, and the other ingredients, toss, put the lid on, and cook on Low for 7 hours.

2.Divide the mix between plates and serve right away.

Nutrition: 241 calories,31.3g protein, 5.4g carbohydrates, 10.8g fat, 1.2g fiber, 81mg cholesterol, 225mg sodium, 550mg potassium.

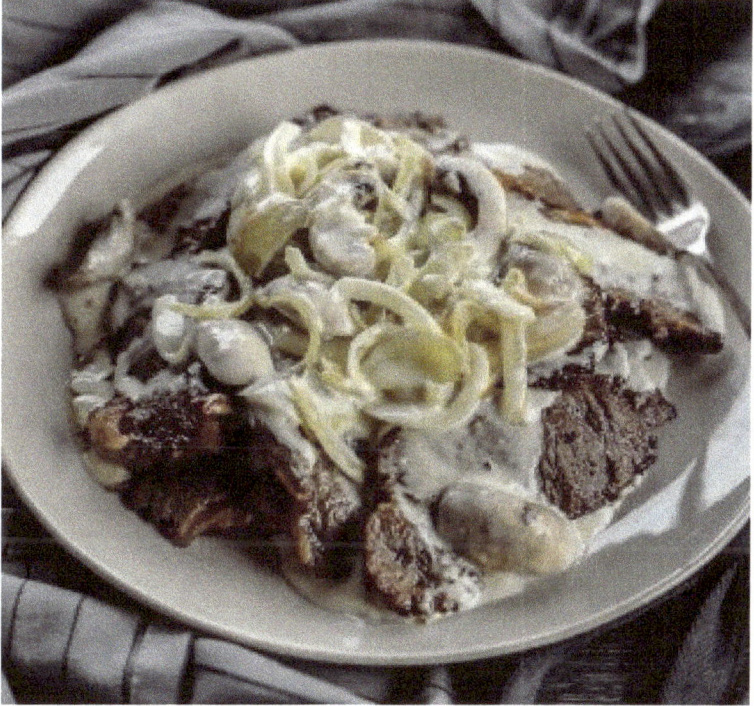

Rosemary Beef with Scallions

Prep Time:
10 minutes
Cook Time:
4 hours
Serve: 4

Ingredients:

- 1 pound beef chops
- 1 tablespoon olive oil
- 3 garlic cloves, minced
- 1 tablespoon rosemary, chopped
- 1 cup kalamata olives, pitted and halved
- 3 scallions, chopped
- 1 teaspoon turmeric powder
- 1 cup beef stock

Directions:

1.In your slow cooker, mix the beef chops with the oil, rosemary, and the other ingredients, toss, put the lid on and cook on High for 4 hours.

2.Divide the mix between plates and serve.

Nutrition: 386 calories,23.5g protein, 4.6g carbohydrates, 30.5g fat, 1.9g fiber, 85mg cholesterol, 547mg sodium, 97mg potassium.

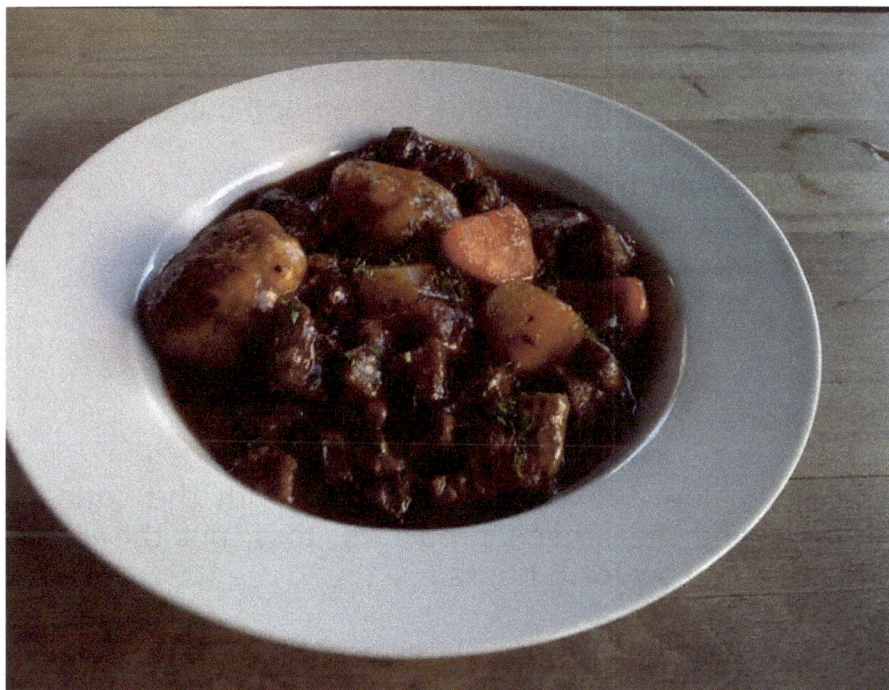

Nutmeg Beef

Prep Time:
10 minutes
Cook Time:
6 hours
 Serve: 4

Ingredients:

- 1 pound beef loin, roughly cubed
- 1 cup butternut squash, peeled and cubed
- ½ teaspoon nutmeg, ground
- ½ teaspoon chili powder
- ½ teaspoon coriander, ground
- 2 teaspoons olive oil
- 1 cup beef stock
- 1 tablespoon cilantro, chopped

Directions:

1.In your slow cooker, mix the beef with the squash, nutmeg, and the other ingredients, toss, put the lid on and cook on Low for 6 hours.

2.Divide the mix between plates and serve.

Nutrition: 249 calories,31.4g protein, 4.4g carbohydrates, 12.1g fat, 0.9g fiber, 81mg cholesterol, 263mg sodium, 549mg potassium.

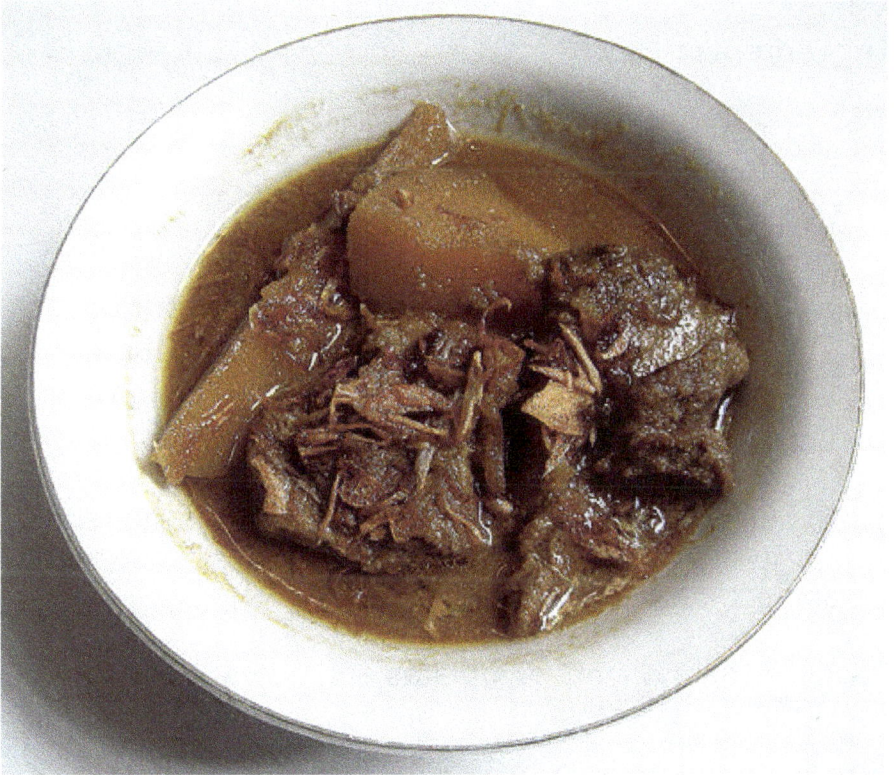

Aromatic Fennel Beef

Prep Time:
10 minutes
Cook Time:
 4 hours
Serve: 4

Ingredients:

- 1 pound beef loin, roughly cubed
- 1 fennel bulb, sliced
- 1 tablespoon lemon juice
- 1 teaspoon avocado oil
- ½ teaspoon coriander, ground
- 1 cup tomato passata
- 1 tablespoon cilantro, chopped

Directions:

1.In your slow cooker, combine the beef with the fennel, lemon juice, and the other ingredients, toss, put the lid on and cook on High for 4 hours.

2.Divide the mix between plates and serve.

Nutrition: 235 calories,31.5g protein, 6g carbohydrates, 9.8g fat, 1.9g fiber, 81mg cholesterol, 94mg sodium, 636mg potassium.

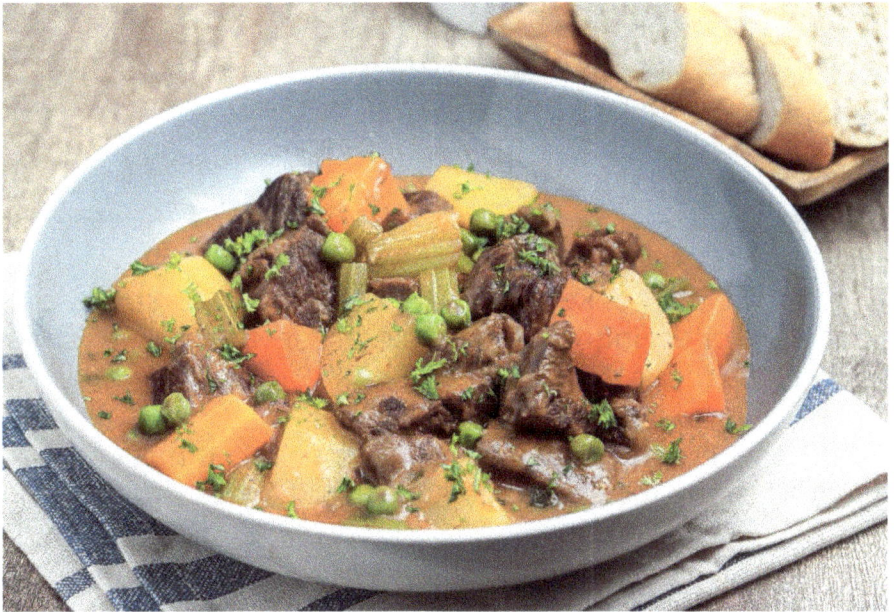

Creamy Beef with Turmeric

Prep Time:
10 minutes
Cook Time:
6 hours
Serve: 4

- 2 pounds beef loin, cubed
- 1 cup Greek-style yogurt
- 1/3 cup beef stock
- 2 teaspoons avocado oil
- 1 teaspoon turmeric powder
- 1 red onion, sliced
- 1 tablespoon cilantro, chopped

Directions:

1.In your slow cooker, mix the beef with the stock, oil, and the other ingredients except for the greek style yogurt, toss, put the lid on, and cook on Low for 5 hours.

2.Add the cream, toss, cook on Low for 1 more hour, divide the mix into bowls and serve.

Nutrition: 470 calories,67g protein, 5.4g carbohydrates, 20.1g fat, 0.8g fiber, 166mg cholesterol, 216mg sodium, 918mg potassium.

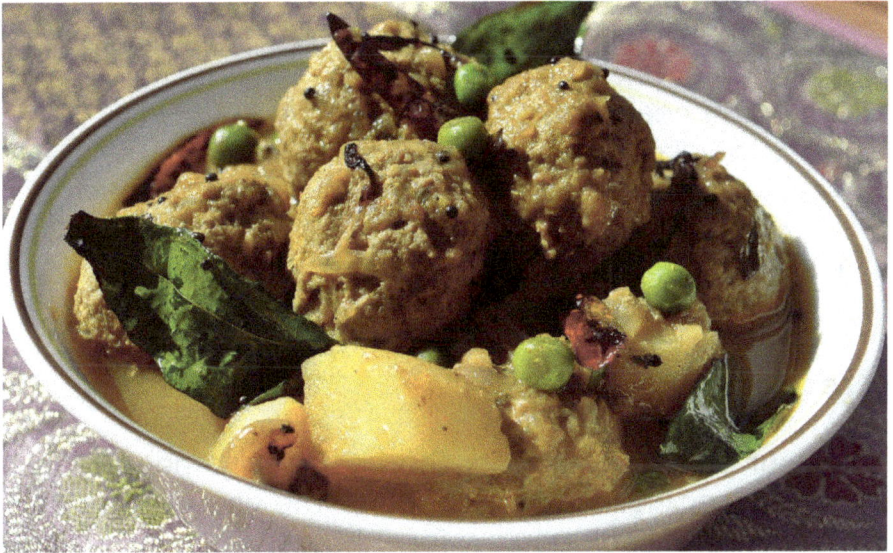

Beef with Capers

Prep Time:
10 minutes
Cook Time:
7 hours
Serve: 4

Ingredients:

- 1 pound beef loin, cubed
- 1 tablespoon capers, drained
- 1 cup greek style yogurt
- ½ cup beef stock
- ½ tablespoon mustard
- 3 scallions, chopped
- 2 teaspoons avocado oil
- 1 teaspoon cumin, ground
- 1 tablespoon parsley, chopped

Directions:

1.In your slow cooker, mix the beef with capers, stock, and the other ingredients except for the yogurt, toss, put the lid on, and cook on Low for 6 hours.

2.Add the yogurt, toss, cook on Low for 1 more hour, divide the mix between plates and serve.

Nutrition: 258 calories,32.4g protein, 4.9g carbohydrates, 12.3g fat, 0.8g fiber, 81mg cholesterol, 237mg sodium, 460mg potassium.

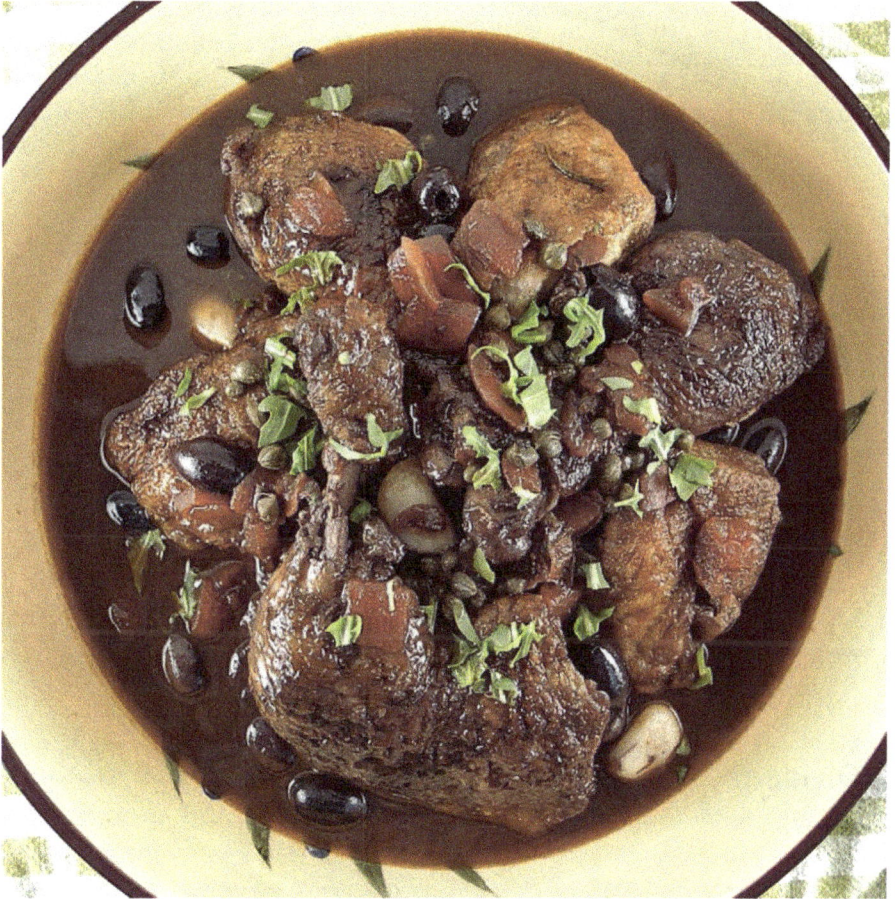

Masala Beef

Prep Time:
10 minutes
Cook Time:
7 hours
Serve: 4

Ingredients:

- 1 pound beef loin, cubed
- 1 teaspoon garam masala
- 1 tablespoon olive oil
- 1 tablespoon lime zest, grated
- 1 tablespoon lime juice
- ½ teaspoon sweet paprika
- ½ teaspoon coriander, ground
- 1 cup beef stock

Directions:

1.In your slow cooker, mix the beef with the garam masala, oil, and the other ingredients, toss, put the lid on and cook on Low for 7 hours.

2.Divide the mix between plates and serve.

Nutrition: 244 calories,31.1g protein, 0.9g carbohydrates, 13.1g fat, 0.3g fiber, 81mg cholesterol, 260mg sodium, 432mg potassium.

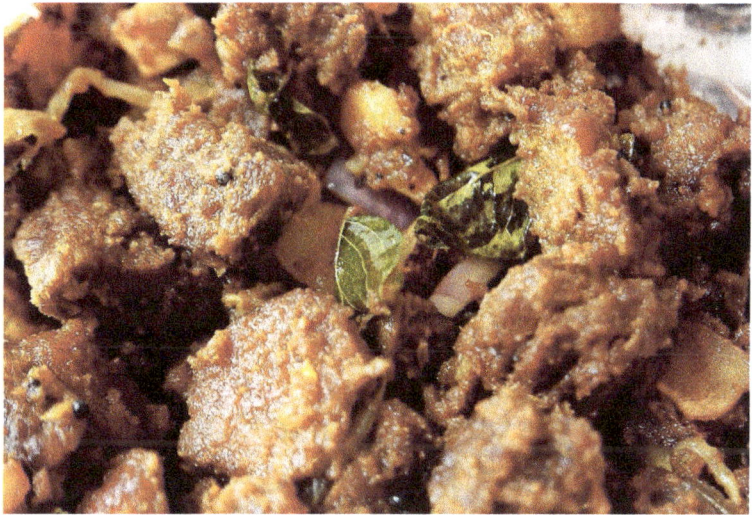

Cabbage and Beef Saute

Prep Time:
10 minutes
Cook Time:
5 hours
Serve: 8

Ingredients:

- 2 pounds beef loin, cubed
- 1 cup red cabbage, shredded
- 1 cup beef stock
- 1 teaspoon avocado oil
- 1 teaspoon sweet paprika
- 2 tablespoons tomato paste
- 1 tablespoon cilantro, chopped

Directions:

1.In your slow cooker, mix the beef with the cabbage, stock, and the other ingredients, toss, put the lid on and cook on High for 5 hours.

2.Divide everything between plates and serve.

Nutrition: 216 calories,31g protein, 1.5g carbohydrates, 9.7g fat, 0.5g fiber, 81mg cholesterol, 166mg sodium, 466mg potassium.

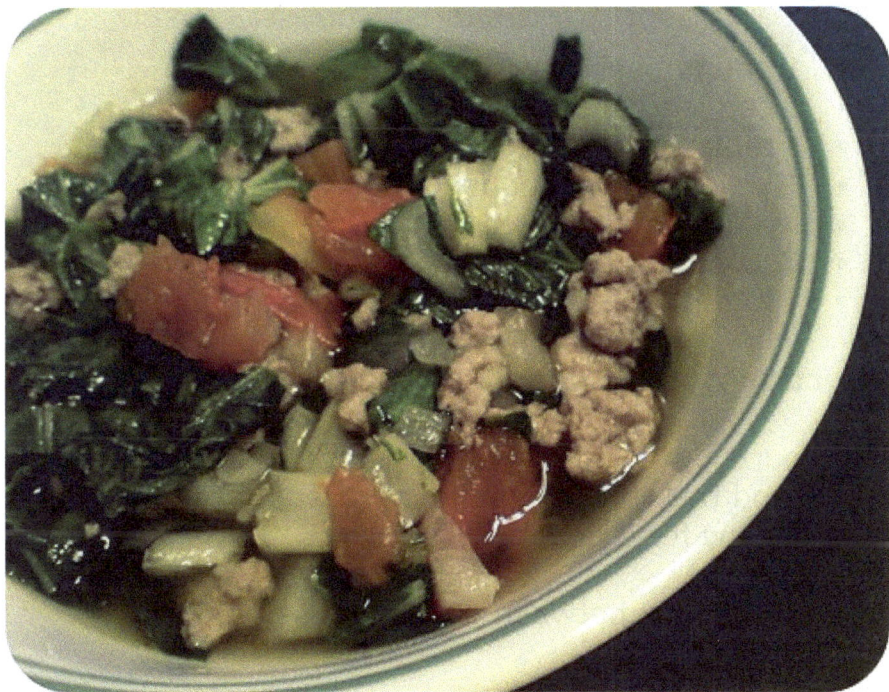

Tender Beef with Lentils

Prep Time:
10 minutes
Cook Time:
7 hours
Serve: 4

Ingredients:

- 1 pound beef loin, cubed
- 1 cup lentils, drained and rinsed, cooked
- 1 tablespoon olive oil
- 1 yellow onion, chopped
- ¼ cup tomato sauce
- ¼ cup beef stock
- 1 tablespoon cilantro, chopped

Directions:

1.In your slow cooker, mix the beef with the lentils, oil, onion, and the other ingredients, toss, put the lid on and cook on Low for 7 hours.

2.Divide the mix between plates and serve.

Nutrition: 423 calories,44.3g protein, 32.3g carbohydrates, 13.6g fat, 15.5g fiber, 81mg cholesterol, 196mg sodium, 944mg potassium.

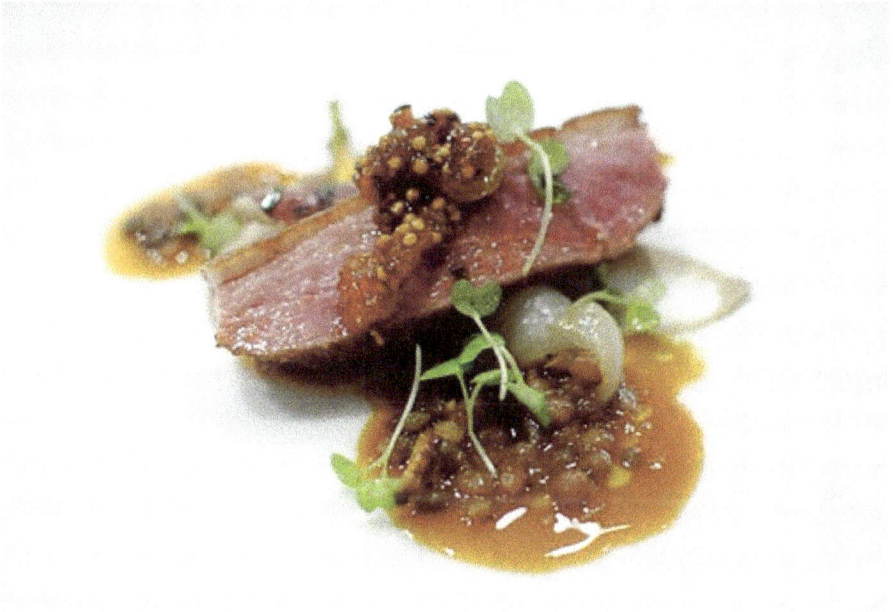

Coriander Beef Mix

Prep Time:
10 minutes
Cook Time:
7 hours
Serve: 4

Ingredients:

- 1 pound beef loin, cubed
- 2 teaspoons avocado oil
- 1 tablespoon balsamic vinegar
- ½ teaspoon coriander, ground
- 1 cup beef stock

Directions:

1.In your slow cooker, mix the beef with the oil, vinegar, and the other ingredients, toss, put the lid on and cook on Low for 7 hours.

2.Divide the mix between plates and serve with a side salad.

Nutrition: 214 calories,31g protein, 0.2g carbohydrates, 9.9g fat, 0.1g fiber, 81mg cholesterol, 258mg sodium, 428mg potassium.

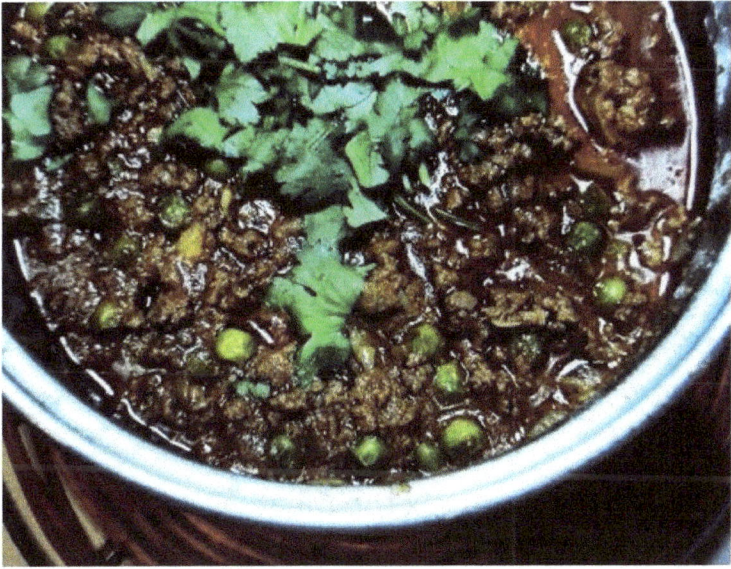

Beef and Endives Bowls

Prep Time:
10 minutes
Cook Time:
7 hours
Serve: 4

Ingredients:

- 1 pound beef loin, cubed
- 2 teaspoons avocado oil
- 2 endives, shredded
- ½ cup beef stock
- ½ teaspoon sweet paprika
- ¼ cup tomato passata
- 3 garlic cloves, minced
- 1 tablespoon chives, chopped

Directions:

1.In your slow cooker, mix the meat with the oil, endives, and the other ingredients, toss, put the lid on and cook on Low for 7 hours.

2.Divide the mix between plates and serve.

Nutrition: 261 calories,34.2g protein, 10g carbohydrates, 10.4g fat, 8.2g fiber, 81mg cholesterol, 217mg sodium, 1232mg potassium.

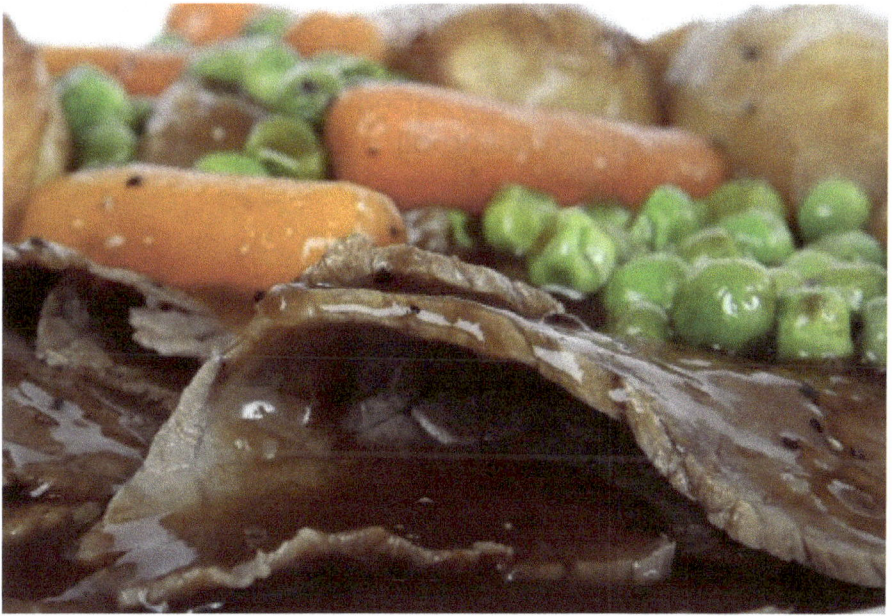

Beef and Lime

Prep Time:
10 minutes
Cook Time:
4 hours
Serve: 4

Ingredients:

- 1 pound beef loin, roughly cubed
- 2 small zucchinis, cubed
- Juice of 1 lime
- ½ teaspoon rosemary, dried
- 2 tablespoons avocado oil
- 1 red onion, chopped
- ½ cup beef stock
- 1 tablespoon garlic, minced
- 1 tablespoon cilantro, chopped

Directions:

1.In your slow cooker, mix the beef with the zucchinis, lime juice, and the other ingredients, toss, put the lid on and cook on High for 4 hours.

2.Divide the mix between plates and serve.

Nutrition: 242 calories,31.9g protein, 5.8g carbohydrates, 10.6g fat, 1.7g fiber, 81mg cholesterol, 168mg sodium, 630mg potassium.

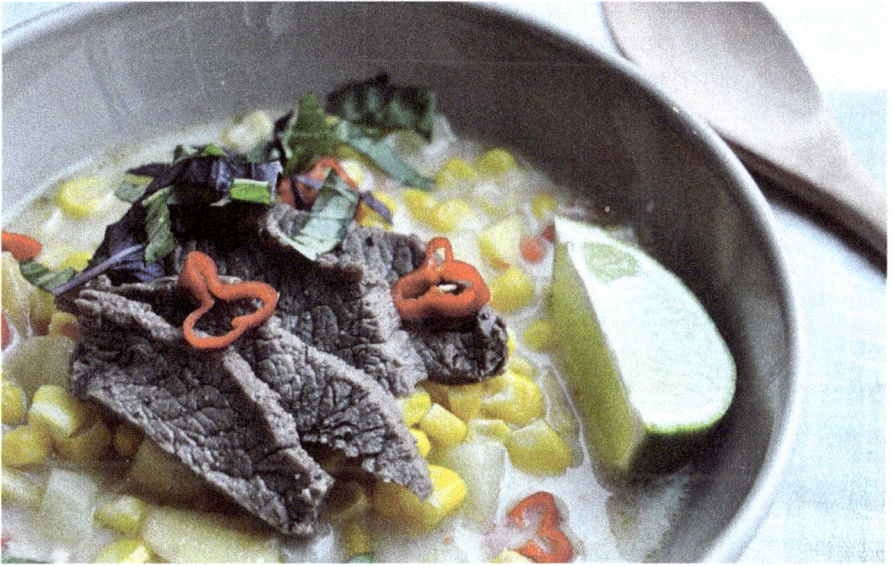

Beef Curry with Mustard

Prep Time:
10 minutes
Cook Time:
8 hours
Serve: 8

Ingredients:

- 2 pounds beef steak, cubed
- 2 tablespoons olive oil
- 3 potatoes, diced
- 1 tablespoon mustard
- 2 ½ tablespoons curry powder
- 2 yellow onions, chopped
- 2 garlic cloves, minced
- 10 ounces of coconut milk
- 2 tablespoons tomato sauce

Directions:

1.In your Slow cooker, mix oil with steak, potatoes, mustard, curry powder, garlic, coconut milk, tomato sauce, pepper, toss, cover, and cook on Low for 8 hours.

2.Stir curry one more time, divide into bowls and serve.

Nutrition: 403 calories,37.6g protein, 19.2g carbohydrates, 19.8g fat, 4.2g fiber, 101mg cholesterol, 107mg sodium, 971mg potassium.

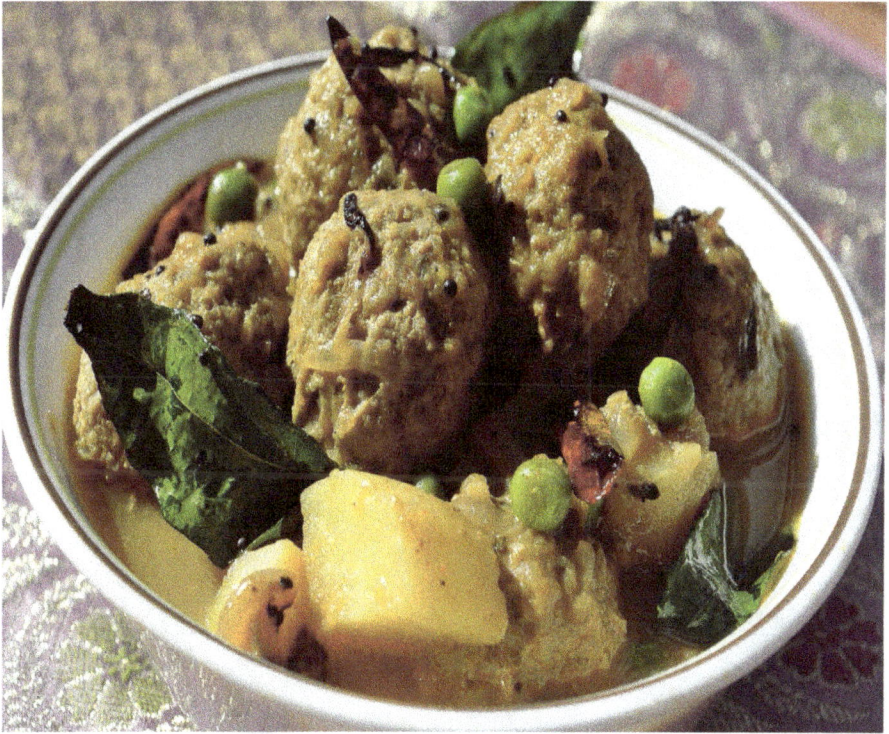

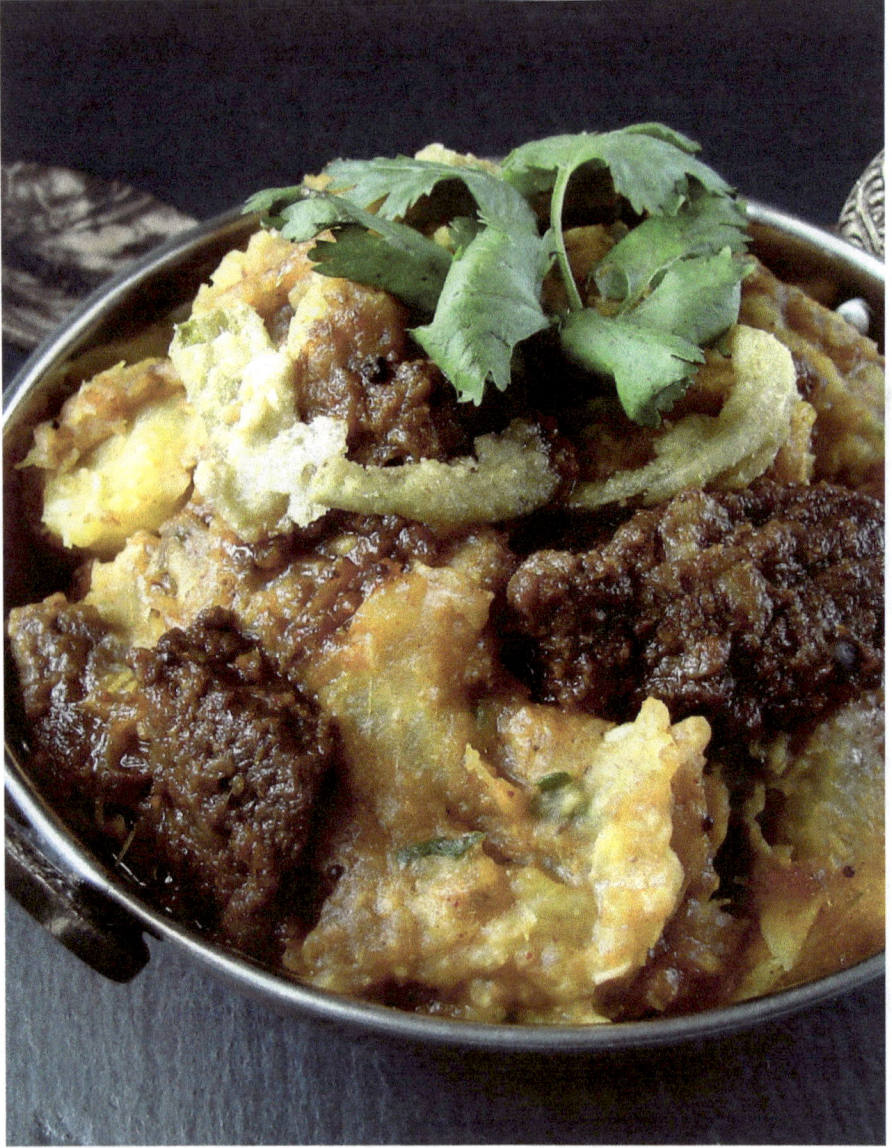

www.ingramcontent.com/pod-product-compliance
Lightning Source LLC
Chambersburg PA
CBHW062343300326
41947CB00012B/1190